THE HISTORY OF MEDICINE SERIES
ISSUED UNDER THE AUSPICES
OF THE LIBRARY OF THE
NEW YORK ACADEMY OF MEDICINE

No. 40

Documents and Dates of Modern Discoveries in the Nervous System

[by Alexander Walker]

A facsimile of the original edition, London, 1839,
with an introduction

by

PAUL F. CRANEFIELD

Published under the auspices of The Library of
The New York Academy of Medicine

Scarecrow Reprint Corporation
Metuchen, N.J. 1973

Documents and Dates of Modern Discoveries in the Nervous System is reprinted from the original edition published in 1839 by John Churchill in London. The copy used in preparing this reprint is from the collection of The Library of The New York Academy of Medicine.

Library of Congress Cataloging in Publication Data

Walker, Alexander, physiologist.
Documents and dates of modern discoveries in the nervous system.

(The History of medicine series, no. 40)
A facism. of the original 1839 ed. published by J. Churchill, London; with new introd.
"Published under the auspices of the Library of the New York Academy of Medicine."
Bibliography: p.
1. Nervous system. I. New York Academy of Medicine. Library. II. Title. III. Series.
QP361.W36 1839a 612'.819 73-9860
ISBN 0-8108-0664-9

INTRODUCTION

IN 1809 Alexander Walker suggested that the roots of the spinal nerves differ in function, the anterior root being sensory and the dorsal root being motor. This erroneous idea gained Walker a permanent if somewhat curious place in the history of science since it linked his name to the important discovery of the actual state of affairs, namely that the dorsal root is sensory and that the anterior root is motor. I have reviewed elsewhere the claims of Walker, Charles Bell and François Magendie to priority in that discovery (Cranefield, 1973). My conclusions, in brief, are that Walker was the first to conjecture that one root is sensory and the other motor, whereas Magendie was the first to assign the functions correctly and to offer definitive experimental evidence proving that the anterior root is motor and that the dorsal root is sensory.

Walker, however, never relinquished his original opinion and maintained to the end of his life that the anterior root is sensory and the dorsal, motor. He was thereby led into a long polemic in support of two claims: first, that he had been deprived of credit for his great discovery; and second, that his great discovery had not only been "borrowed" from him but had been "inverted." Walker thus claimed that Bell and Magendie had stolen the credit from him and gotten the facts wrong to boot.

Walker's defense of his priority was developed at great length in two books. One was his *The nervous system . . .* (1834); the other was the volume here reprinted in facsimile, the anonymous *Documents and dates of modern discoveries in the nervous system* (1839). Although this work is anonymous it has always been taken for granted that it is by Walker, and there is not the slightest reason to doubt that assumption.

Were Walker's *Documents and dates* . . . merely the ravings of an eccentric anatomist, it might be regarded as an amusing curiosity hardly worth reprinting. It is, however, an important document in the history of the Bell-Magendie controversy. Bell's only claim to priority over Magendie rested on certain half-truths announced in his privately printed and privately circulated pamphlet of 1811, the famous *Idea of a new anatomy of the brain.* Bell and his brothers-in-law, John and Alexander Shaw, quoted passages from the *Idea* in their polemics against Magendie but took care never to reprint the pamphlet in its entirety. It was Walker's *Documents and dates* that made Bell's *Idea* available to the public for the first time. (Bell's *Idea* was never published by Bell himself. Its first appearance, in 1811, was as a privately printed and privately circulated edition of 100 copies; its second appearance was in 1812 when it was reprinted, apparently without Bell's knowledge or consent, in the *Baltimore Medical and Philosophical Lycaeum* 1:303-318, 1811 [actually 1812]; its third appearance was in Walker's *Documents and dates* . . .; and it was first "officially" published long after Bell's death when Bell's brother-in-law, Alexander Shaw, with the consent of Bell's widow, reprinted it in 1869 in the *Journal of Anatomy and Physiology*, 3:147-182. Full details of this curious series of events are found in Cranefield, 1973.)

Walker's *Documents and dates*... contains, however, much more than Bell's *Idea.* It contains excerpts from his own work and it contains the original French texts and excellent translations of Magendie's articles on the nerve roots. Moreover, the second half of *Documents and dates* contains an admirable collection of excerpts from articles dealing with the then very recent discovery of the spinal reflex, a discovery that had already generated a priority controversy as ugly as that between Bell and Magendie. In the controversy over the discovery of the spinal reflex the injured party was, of course, Marshall Hall.

Walker's *Documents and dates* . . . thus merits reprinting because it is a fascinating document in itself, because of its historical importance in making Bell's *Idea* generally available for the first time, because it contains a still useful collection of texts on the discovery of the function of the spinal nerve roots, and because it contains an interesting and very early collection of texts on the discovery of the spinal reflex.

Not a great deal is known of Walker's life. A short sketch given by Struthers (1867, pp. 76-78) follows:

"Alexander Walker is better known as an author than as a lecturer. He published the following works [Struther here lists Walker's *Physiognomy . . .*, *The nervous system . . .*, *Beauty . . .*, *Intermarriage . . .*, *Documents and dates . . .*, *Woman . . .*, and *Pathology . . .*, for which see bibliography].

"Mr. Walker was born 20th December 1779. He had worked at anatomy with Dr. Barclay, and at the age of twenty went to London, where he continued his anatomical pursuits. Returning to Edinburgh about 1808, he gave lectures in the Lyceum and elsewhere, which were numerously attended by students and medical practitioners. He also gave lectures in the Assembly Rooms, to mixed audiences, 'On general and particular science.' I am uncertain how far his lectures in Edinburgh were regular courses or special and fragmentary. He attracted considerable notice by instructing the students as to the mode of cutting down on arteries, for which he gave exact mathematical directions. In London he had had to leave the school in consequence of showing the students, after lecture, that Abernethy, instead of tying the subclavian artery, had put the ligature round the neighboring nerve-trunk. What position he had occupied at St. Bartholomew's, or in Abernethy's class, I am unaware, but the incident of the nerve being tied instead of the artery (on the dead subject), and Mr. Walker's giving offence and having to leave there, in consequence of pointing it out, I have on good authority. After a few years he returned to London, where his career was mostly literary. He was connected with several newspapers, was an active founder of the *Literary Gazette*, and published the contributions to science and art above enumerated. He had not, so far as I am aware, graduated, or desired to graduate, in medicine or surgery, although he worked at anatomy. He returned to Edinburgh in 1842, in weak health, and died Dec. 6, 1852, in his seventy-third year.

"There is considerable merit and originality in some of Mr.

Walker's views, especially in regard to the cerebellum. I saw him often in his later years, when he resided in the neighbourhood of Leith, and was under the friendly professional care of my brother Dr. James Struthers. Although his faculties had become considerably impaired, he was able to converse regarding his views on the nervous system, and still maintained to me that Bell was wrong, that the posterior root is the motor, and the anterior the sensory root. Tracing the connexion between the cerebellum and the posterior column of the spinal cord, he inferred, from the views he held regarding the cerebellum, that the posterior root of the spinal nerve must be motor, leaving the sensory function to the anterior root. His claims to priority in the idea of the two roots having distinct functions are fully discussed in his work on the Nervous System."

To this sketch I can add that one of Walker's earliest works, his *Outline of a natural system of medical science* (1808) is polemical in tone and eccentric in style, so that we need not assume that either quality grew out of his having became embittered by his role in the discovery of the function of the roots of the spinal nerves. Nor should one overlook, in all the polemic and eccentricity, the fact that Walker had a brilliant mind and a wry sense of humor and appears to have begun life as a first rate anatomist, while the many editions of his popular books testify to his skill as a writer.

Paul F. Cranefield
The Rockefeller University
New York, New York

BIBLIOGRAPHY

Charles Bell. *Idea of a new anatomy of the brain.* n.p., n.d.[London Strahan and Preston, 1811.]

Paul F. Cranefield. *The way in and the way out. François Magendie, Charles Bell and the roots of the spinal nerves.* In press.

John Struthers. *Historical sketch of the Edinburgh anatomical school.* Edinburgh, Maclachlan and Stewart, 1867.

The following list of Walker's publications is probably far from complete; moreover many of the entries are taken from secondary sources. The first and second entries *(Anatomia Britannica)* are probably not by Walker at all; they were, however, attributed to him during his life time (see *British and Foreign Medical Review* 9:118n, 1840). The list is based on copies I have seen and on copies listed in the catalogues or printed catalogues of the British Museum (BM), The New York Academy of Medicine (NYAM), The Wellcome Medical Historical Institute (W), Edinburgh University (E), National Library of Medicine *(Index Catalogue)* (NLM), the Library of Congress (LC) and *The Royal Society Catalogue of Scientific Papers* (RSC). An entry that ends with an asterisk refers to a copy I have seen. Since some of the works are rare and no library contains all of them I have listed at the end of entries for the less common items the libraries whose catalogues contain these works.

Anonymous [Alexander Walker??] *Anatomia Britannica. A system of anatomy and physiology selected from the works of Haller, Albinus, Monro, Winslow, Hunter, Soemmerring, Scarpa, Cruikshank, Masgagni, Murray, Walter, Sabatier, Meckel, Zinn, etc. etc. etc.* London, J. Scott, 1804.* [E]

Anonymous [Alexander Walker??] *Anatomia Britannica. A system of anatomy and physiology . . .* 2nd ed., London, Thomas Wilson, 1808* [E,W,NLM]

Alexander Walker. *Prospectus of two courses of lectures: one on anatomy and physiology; the other on pathology and the practice of medicine.* Edinburgh, University Press, 1808. [NLM]

Alexander Walker. *Prospectus of lectures on the natural system of universal science.* n.p. n.d. [Edinburgh, 1808?]. [E]

Alexander Walker. *Tables of a Natural System of Medical Science.* Edinburgh, Oliver and Boyd, 1808. [W]

Alexander Walker. *Outline of a natural system of medical science. Forming the preliminary lectures to two courses: one on anatomy and physiology; the other on pathology and the practice of medicine.* Edinburgh, Prined [sic] at the University Press. For Sir Richard Phillips, No. 6 Brigde-Street, Blackfriars, London, and Messrs. T. Bryce and Co. Infirmary-Street, Edinburgh, 1808.* [NLM]

Alexander Walker. *Result of the operation, publicly performed in order to refute or to confirm the principle of surgical operation proposed by . . .* Edinburgh, R. Phillips, 1808.* [NLM]

Alexander Walker. Theory of phonics, hearing, &c. Physiological dissertation on the functions of the Ossicula auditus, and on the tympanic muscles in particular, and on those of the ear in general. *London Med. and Phys. Journ.* 19:385-414, 1808. [Cited from RSC]

Alexander Walker, editor, *Archives of Universal Science,* vols. 1, 2, 3. Edinburgh, 1809.* [W,BM]

Alexander Walker. Preliminary Discourse. *Archives of Universal Science,* 1:i-xl, 1809.*

Alexander Walker. General physiology of the intellectual organs. *Archives of Universal Science,* 2:167-205, 1809.*

Alexander Walker. New anatomy and physiology of the brain in particular, and of the nervous system in general. *Archives of Universal Science,* 3:172-179, 1809.*

Alexander Walker. On the use of the cerebellum and spinal marrow. *Annals of Philosophy,* 5:316-317, 1815.*

Alexander Walker. Sketch of a general theory of the intellectual functions of man and animals given in reply to Drs. Cross and Leach. *Annals of Philosophy,* 6:26-34 and 118-124, 1815.*

Alexander Walker. A simple theory of Electricity and Galvanism, being an attempt to prove that the subjects of the former are the mere oxygen and azote of the air, and the subjects of the latter the mere oxygen and hydrogen of water. *Annals of Philosophy*, 8:182-189, 1816. [Cited from RSC]

Alexander Walker. On the cause of the directions of continents and islands, peninsulas, mountains, chains, strata, currents, winds, migrations, and civilization. *Phil. Mag.* 3:426-431, 1833. [Cited from RSC, a typical Walker title but I have not ascertained whether this article is by "the" Alexander Walker.]

Alexander Walker. *The nervous system, anatomical and physiological; in which the functions of the various parts of the brain are for the first time assigned; and to which is prefixed some account of the author's earliest discoveries, of which the more recent doctrine of Bell, Magendie, etc., is shewn to be at once a plagiarism, an inversion, and a blunder, associated with useless experiments which they have neither understood nor explained. Being the first volume of an original system of physiology, adapted to the advanced state of anatomy.* London, Smith, Elder & Co., 1834.* [W, NLM, NYAM]

Alexander Walker. *Physiognomy founded on physiology and applied to various countries, professions and individuals; with an appendix on the bones at Hythe, the sculls of the ancient inhabitants of Britain and its invaders.* London, Smith, Elder & Co., 1834. [NLM, NYAM]

Alexander Walker. *Beauty; illustrated chiefly by an analysis and classification of beauty in woman. Preceded by a critical view of the general hypotheses respecting beauty, by Hume, Hogarth, Burke, Knight, Alison, etc., and followed by a similar view of the hypotheses of beauty in sculpture and painting, by Leonardo da Vinci, Winckelmann, Mengs, Bossi, etc.* By Alexander Walker . . . Illustrated by drawings from life, by Henry Howard . . . drawn on stone by M. Gauci and R. J. Lane . . . London, E Wilson, 1836

——,——, New York, W. H. Colyer, 1844.

——,——, 2nd ed., London, H. G. Bohn, 1846.

——,——, Hartford, S. Andrus & Son, 1851.

——,——, London, H. G. Bohn, 1852.

——,——, Hartford, S. Andrus & Son, 1854.*

——,——, fifth edition, Glasgow, T. D. Morison, 1892.*

Alexander Walker. *Influence of natural beauty, and of its defects,* *on offspring; and law regulating the resemblance of progeny to parents.* (Pamphlet). London, Stewart & Co., 1837.* [NLM, NYAM]

Alexander Walker. *Intermarriage; or the mode in which, and the causes why, beauty, health and intellect, result from certain unions, and deformity, disease and insanity, from others . . .* London: J. Churchill, 1838.*

——, ——, New York, J. & H. G. Langley, 1839.*

——, ——, 2nd edition, London, J. Churchill, 1841.

——, ——, 2nd edition, New York, J. & H. G. Langley, 1842.*

——, ——, Philadelphia, Lindsay & Blakiston, 1853.*

——, ——, Philadelphia, Lindsay & Blakiston, 1860.*

——, ——, Philadelphia, Lindsay & Blakiston, 1866.

——, ——, Birmingham [England], Edward Baker, 1897.

Alexander Walker. *Woman physiologically considered as to mind, morals, marriage, matrimonial slavery, infidelity, and divorce.* London, 1839.

——, ——, New York, J. & H. G. Langley, 1840.

——, ——, 2nd ed., London, A. H. Baily, 1840.*

——, ——, new ed., Hartford, S. Andrus & Son, 1851.

——, ——, Birmingham [England], E. Baker, 1898.

Anonymous [Alexander Walker]. *Documents and Dates of Modern Discoveries in the Nervous System.* London, Churchill, 1839.*

Alexander Walker. *The new Lavater: a system of physiognomy, founded upon strictly scientific principles . . . To which are added, remarks on phrenology, etc.* London, 1839. [E]

Alexander Walker. *Pathology, founded on the natural system of anatomy and physiology; a philosophical sketch, in which the natural classification of diseases, and the distinction between morbid and curative symptoms, afforded by pain or its absence, are pointed out; as well as the errors of homoeopathy and other hypotheses.* 2 ed. London, J. Churchill, 1841.

——, ——, New York, J. & H. G. Langley, 1842.

Alexander Walker. Purification of Edinburgh, etc. [Letters on the sanitary condition of Edinburgh.] [Edinburgh, 1842.] [BM]

Alexander Walker. *The anthropological works of Alexander Walker.* 3 v. New ed. New York, J. & H. G. Langley, 1843. Contents:

v. 1. Beauty, illustrated chiefly by an analysis and classification of beauty in women.

v. 2. Intermarriage, or the mode in which, and the causes why, beauty, health and intellect, result from certain unions, and deformity, disease, and insanity from others; demonstrated by delineations of the structure and forms, and descriptions of the functions and capacities, which each parent, in every pair, bestows on children, in conformity with certain natural laws, and by an account of corresponding effects in the breeding of animals.

v. 3. Women physiologically considered, as to mind, morals, marriage, matrimonial slavery, infidelity and divorce. With an appendix, containing notes and additions. Edited by an American physician.

Alexander Walker. *The book of beauty; with modes for improving and preserving it in man and woman. As also for beautifying the shape and attitude and maintaining the appearance of youth till past middle age. In which is included advice on the art of dressing, showing the styles and colors of costume most becoming to the various sizes, complexions and forms of the human race.* By Alexander Walker. From the 5th London ed. New York, Holland & Glover, 1843. [LC]

Alexander Walker. *Female beauty. Being a complete analysis and description of every part of woman's form, and showing her perfect capacities for the purposes of love; procreative duties and happiness* . . . New York, J. H. Farrell, 1856(?). [LC]

DOCUMENTS AND DATES

OF

MODERN DISCOVERIES

IN THE

NERVOUS SYSTEM.

On every subject of the work, the Editor is desirous of avoiding all expression of his own opinion, when it can be supposed to have the slightest relation to any of the Authors of these discoveries.

INTRODUCTORY REMARKS.

LONDON:

JOHN CHURCHILL, PRINCE'S STREET, SOHO.

MDCCCXXXIX.

LONDON:
PRINTED BY STEWART AND MURRAY,
OLD BAILEY.

CONTENTS, WITH DATES OF DOCUMENTS.

ADVERTISEMENT.

WITH a knowledge of the transcendent importance of the subjects of these Papers, the frequency and the heat of contests as to priority of discovery, both in England and on the Continent, appear to have increased. To restore peace, in this respect, to the republic of science, the Editor has supposed that nothing could so much contribute, as a concentrated view of Documents and Dates.

These documents will be the more valuable, that some of them cannot now be purchased.—To confer on them the highest degree of authenticity, every paper originally published in a foreign language, is printed in that language, as well as in English.—To save trouble to the reader, all irrelevant matter is carefully rejected: but not one word is omitted that bears on the proper subject of the paper.—To permit the more easy formation of opinion, the passages in each that are clearly fundamental, are marked by small capitals, or by italics.

That these documents are accurately inserted, and that their dates are correct, reference to any one of the originals which may happen to be within reach of a reader, will give indisputable evidence. The

Editor aspires only to the thanks due to absolute impartiality and scrupulous accuracy.

A physiologist has suggested the arrangement of this work according to the classes of organs composing the NERVOUS SYSTEM. The following is the reasoning he employs:

There are THREE DISTINCT CLASSES OF ORGANS IN THAT SYSTEM—*the higher or mental nervous organs,* of which the centre is in the HEAD; *the intermediate or alternating* nervous organs,* of which the centre is within the SPINE; and *the lower or vital nervous organs,* of which the centres are in the GANGLIA.

The classes of functions are the same in number. *Conscious and voluntary motion* is exercised so long as the CEREBRUM and CEREBELLUM remain; *the greater motions* which alternate—*which may, or may not, be conscious and voluntary,* are exercised so long as the SPINAL MARROW remains; and *the less motions* (those ascribed to irritability), *which are neither conscious nor voluntary,* are exercised after all these organs are destroyed, and while GANGLIA and their nerves alone exist, and chiefly supply the irritable parts,—many of their fibrils being distributed to mere mucous membranes in which none but the minute motions of nutrition and secretion can take place.

The mental nervous organs, then, are distinguished by their acts being subject to consciousness and volition; the vital nervous organs, by their being subject to neither of these; and the intermediate ner-

* The reason for these epithets will speedily appear.

vous organs, by alternating or readily passing from one to the other of these states. Notwithstanding even this capability of transition, all of them are marked by great natural distinctness,—a circumstance essential to the absence of a perpetual substitution of one act for another, and of utter confusion in functional operations.

The functions of these classes of organs, however, have not been sufficiently distinguished by physiologists. Prochaska confounds the greater combined involuntary motions, which belong to the intermediate or spinal organs, with the lesser involuntary motions which belong to the vital or ganglionic organs—acts of deglutition, respiration, &c. with those of peristaltic motion, pulsation, &c. And Mr. Grainger seems to think that "the sympathetic is a part of the excito-motory system," and that "the nervous agency in the two cases is identical." Under reflex function of the spinal marrow, he includes "the contraction exercised by every organ, which produces perceptible motion; whether a muscle of the extremities, the heart, the muscular coat of the intestines, the fibrous tunics of the blood-vessels, or of the secreting canals in glands; in fact, every kind of contraction which is not attributable to elasticity."

Irritation and experiment do not aid us in distinguishing these classes of organs, by displaying their actions. It must be evident to every one, that no actions artificially excited in these organs can possibly resemble their natural ones.—In the higher encephalic organs, in particular, *no voluntary action can be excited at all: force and spontaneity or will are absolutely incompatible:* ALL IRRITATION, THEREFORE, TO COMPEL ANY ACT OF VOLITION, IMPLIES AN ABSURDITY:* this places the first of these classes of organs completely above our reach in experiment.—But *the spinal intermediate or alternating organs are only the complement of the voluntary ones,* assuming and resigning *their* functions at bidding, and always deriving from *them* their principal impulses—their silent guidance: these two classes of organs therefore go together, equally exempt from direct and immediate artificial excitement.—The lower, ganglionic or vital organs may be supposed to be more easily excited to natural action: but their natural excitements are very different from artificial ones—they neither destroy continuity, nor empty the vessels to be actuated. *In all irritations, therefore, even of the lowest and most manageable of these systems, every thing must be forced, perturbed, retrograde—nothing natural, or affording natural conclusion.*

That these classes of nervous organs, moreover, react on each other, we know; as well as that the innumerable accompaniments and terminations of these nerves in the same organs, facilitate this. The higher conscious and voluntary nervous organs, by the

* This presents the remarkable conclusion that *irritation of voluntary parts cannot naturally have* ANY *result.* Irritation has nothing in common with will, and should produce none of its effects.

shocks of emotion and passion, powerfully affect the lower vital and involuntary nervous organs; the vital nervous organs as powerfully affect the two superior classes; and as the highest is untouchable by irritation, it is probably the lowest that, in all that affects life, initiates disturbance. Hence the ease with which irritations of the sympathetic are propagated to the spinal cord, and cause motions in parts deriving nerves from the cerebro-spinal system, as in convulsions in children from intestinal irritation. It must absolutely be on that class of nervous organs alone that all artificial irritation and experiment is *directly* made; and hard must it often be for those who observe not carefully, and reflect not deeply, to tell when its own acts are manifested singly, or when it also drags into its manifestations, acts of the intermediate and alternating, or even of the conscious and voluntary system.

It is easy to say that the actions caused by pricking a divided nerve, tremors, shiverings, twitchings, belong to the ganglionic organs; and that the motions caused by applying stimulants to the skin—combined motions, as those of the limbs in retracting, or as the more general efforts of the whole body—motions having a preservative character, and ceasing when the spinal marrow is removed, belong to the intermediate organs. But these actions pass imperceptibly into each other; and the philosopher who contemplates them will see how much even he has to do before he can, from irritation or experiment, draw any safe inference as to the distinctions and the real nature of these classes of organs.

After what has been said, there is, indeed, little difficulty in distinguishing the mental conscious and voluntary acts from all others. The great difficulty is to distinguish the vital inconscious and involuntary from the intermediate or alternating acts. The following consideration, however, I think affords a test: *The ganglionic nerves are primarily and directly those only of the tubular organs, which transmit and transmute liquids, and constitute the vital system—hence irritation of the cœliac ganglion accelerates the peristaltic motions of the intestines; those actions, therefore, can alone be theirs which naturally and directly affect these organs; and* WHENEVER ANY OF THE STRAIGHT MUSCLES EMPLOYED IN OTHER THAN VITAL ACTS ARE INVOLVED, IT MUST BE BECAUSE THE INTERMEDIATE OR ALTERNATING ORGANS ARE DRAGGED INTO VITAL MANIFESTATIONS.*

Enough, then, appears to show, that it is according to the indications which are here afforded, and which are applicable to still higher objects, that any series of papers on the nervous system should be arranged, so as to afford an enlarged foundation for physiological induction.

* How deserving the epithet of "intermediate or alternating," the spinal organs are, is now evident.

INTRODUCTORY REMARKS.

EVERYWHERE throughout Europe the investigations of anatomists and physiologists are directed to the Nervous System. A greater or more deeply interesting subject it is certainly impossible to imagine; for by knowledge of it alone can humanity be guaranteed against the most frightful diseases,—by it alone can we fulfil the high injunction "Know Thyself,"—by it alone, are laid open to us the philosophy of the mind, and all the profound and beautiful arts that depend on it. It is these high duties and prospects that render medicine the noblest of professions, and its scientific professors the most worthy of human respect.

The ascription of sensitive functions to one of the two series—to the anterior, or to the posterior series, of cerebral masses, columns of spinal marrow, and nerves attached to them,—the ascription of voluntary functions to the remaining series of cerebral masses, spinal columns and attached nerves,—and a connection through the brain and cerebellum between the anterior and the posterior of these series, forming thereby a circle of nervous action and influence, is the conception of recent times.

The precise direction or course of this action,—whether from the anterior to the posterior series, or vice versa,—whether from before backward, or from behind forward,—has been the great subject of doubt.

This, it was thought, might be determined by experiment. For that purpose, the roots, anterior and posterior, of the spinal nerves, seeing that these were then deemed either purely sensitive or purely motive, were thought to be the only parts at which we could hope that artificial irritations might produce successful results—decisive evidence of the direction and course of the mental functions.

Accordingly, after many experiments on the higher animals, then thought doubtful, such results were, a few years ago, supposed by perhaps the greater number of physiologists, to be yielded by Müller's experiments on frogs, which seemed to indicate motion to be the function of the anterior parts, and sensation to be the function of the posterior ones.

Even *then*, however, it was not forgotten, that the first experiments of Magendie had exhibited motion as the result of irritating either anterior or posterior parts in the HIGHER ANIMALS. *Now*, other circumstances, causing further indecision and doubt, have arisen: the experiments of Hall have proved that motion is produced by irritating either root in LOWER ANIMALS,—turtles and rays. Thus, strangely, is one and the same effect produced by irritating parts which must be directly opposed in function! Finally, the circumstances in the structure of frogs pointed out by Volkmann (an anomalous distribution of ganglia and ganglionic fibrils upon the precise parts which are the subjects of experiment), must, in all experiments on these animals, have been attended by demonstrations only of correspondingly anomalous, instead of regular, function.

Under these circumstances of indecision and doubt as to past experiments—of parts *different* in nature manifesting *similar* results, is this fundamental question again thrown open to discussion.

If, from experiment, we recur to reasoning, *it certainly seems impossible that mental nerves, pure nerves of sensation on one hand, and pure nerves of volition on the other — nerves directly opposed in their nature, as the spinal roots are thus supposed to be, should, on irritation, yield results which are more or less similar, instead of being precisely opposite.*

This brings to recollection, that *both roots are covered by similar ganglionic or vital fibrils;* and it suggests the not illogical conclusion of one of these physiologists, that *that which is similar in the result of these experiments, must be owing, not to that which is different or opposite in the nature of the mental roots themselves, but to that which is similar in the nature of the vital fibrils with which both roots are covered.*

The character, too, of the motions occasioned by such experiments, appears, as observed by the same physiologist, *in no way to resemble that of the calm and deliberate acts induced by impressions on the organ of touch, or of the other mental senses, but that of the involuntary and irresistible spasm or shiver which is always compelled by injury inflicted on the vital nerves, and by the pain which is the outcry of that system when suffering.*

It seems not improbable, therefore, as similarly observed, *that the immediate subject of these experiments has not hitherto been understood; and that, while they have been supposed to be made on the higher, or mental nerves, they have in reality been made on the lower, ganglionic or vital ones, which invest them.*

Unfortunately, these roots are not only undeniably complicated, but it seems quite impossible to separate them into their pure and simple constituent parts—mental roots and ganglionic fibrils—so as to derive from them any satisfactory information by experiment. The law by which nature denies manifestations of sensibility to irritation of the first expansions of the organs of sense, as well as of the brain itself, thus guarding their acts from disturbance, appears to be extended to the least impure of the nerves arising from the spinal marrow. To the interrogation of experiment, we receive from these roots no reply: we hear only the language of the vital nervous system in the expression of pain. Moreover, no cerebral nerve can be proved to be perfectly analogous to any spinal one, and none are much less complicated with ganglionic fibrils.*

If there be no remedy for this, it would seem wise that, in order to unravel the difficulty, physiologists should now rather direct their attention to the structure and the connexion of the parts of the nervous system, to that dependence which such connexion in general very clearly indicates, to the genesis—the successive growth and relative development of parts, to the influences which these point out, and to the beautiful revelations of comparative anatomy.

As a useful preliminary to the future investigation of this great question, it has been thought expedient, at a time when the subject excites such intense and universal attention, to present to the physiological reader a view of its origin in modern times, and of such portion of its progress as renders the state of the question perfectly clear, by laying before him the various documents with their dates, in the precise order in which they originally appeared, without respect to persons, and without a single word of

* There is not the slightest proof that the ganglionic portion of the trifacial, connected with several distinct parts of the brain, and exercising both sensitive and involuntary-motive functions, has any analogy to the posterior roots of the spinal nerves, arising from one and the same part of the spinal cord, and exercising a single function.

comment. These accordingly are here given entire, wherever the subject seemed to require this; and they are abridged only where irrelevant matter had been introduced.

As the subject was investigated in ancient times, however unsuccessfully, it seems advisable to sketch *here* its former progress, instead of making, in the body of the work, a leap of a thousand years in the history of discovery. This procedure is the more expedient, because there is little or no resemblance in ancient and modern notions on the subject. The ancients did suppose a distinction between nerves of sensation and nerves of action; but they had no idea of nerves, spinal columns, and cerebral masses of sensation,—of the continuation of the action thence originating through the cerebrum,—and of other cerebral masses, spinal columns, and nerves of volition, thus forming the great circle of nervous action and influence.

Herophilus and Erasistratus are said to have been the first who distinguished sensitive and motive nerves—*νεῦροι κινητικοὶ* and *νεῦροι αἰσθητικοὶ*, and to have ascribed their difference to this, that the former arose from the substance of the brain, the latter from its membranes. Aretæus made a similar distinction. Rufus Ephesius likewise divided the nerves, which he thought came from the brain, into sentient and moving nerves; Celsus proceeded similarly; but neither, we are told, sufficiently distinguished them from tendons and ligaments! Galen's notions of the nerves, similarly indistinct and inaccurate, descended even to comparatively modern times.

On this subject, as on every other involved in this work, the editor is desirous of avoiding all expression of his own opinion, where it can be supposed to have the slightest relation to any of the authors of these discoveries. Even, therefore, with regard to Galen's doctrines and their bearing on recent ones, he will here quote the language of others.

To the assertion that Galen went even so far as to divide the nerves into nerves of sensation and nerves of motion, Sir C. Bell replies:—"I should have been *proud* to be able to say, that I had reconciled the *theories* of the ancients with the more *perfect knowledge* of modern anatomists; but I *fear* it is not so." "Galen supposed motion and sensation to be the properties of the same nerve, but considered motion to be active and sensation passive, and it was possible, he thought, that there might be nervous power sufficient for sensation, though not for motion. Thus he explained how it happened that sensation remained when motion was lost."*

As giving a more detailed view of this point, the editor quotes the following from a review of Adams's Translation of the Medical Works of Paulus Ægineta, in the Third Number, for April, 1834, of the "Medical Quarterly Review."

"With equal futility Mr. Adams endeavours to give

* The Nervous System, Introduction, p. 4.

to Erasistratus, Aretæus, or Galen, all the merit of *the beautiful modern discovery of the distinct functions of the anterior and posterior columns of the spinal marrow.* In his note on apoplexy and paralysis, in the third book, he makes some more explicit remarks on this subject: —

"'It is impossible to admire too much the brief but comprehensive account of apoplexy and paralysis given by Aretæus. He states decidedly that there is sometimes a loss of motion alone, and sometimes of sensibility; the reason of which he supposes to be that the sensatory and motory nerves are distinct from one another. This is the germ of a theory fully expanded afterwards by Galen, and lately revived by Sir C. Bell, of London, as a new discovery. It appears, indeed, from the anatomical works of Rufus, that the famous Erasistratus had attempted a similar classification of the nerves. Galen, however, has the merit of fully establishing the truth of the theory; and all subsequent writers on physiology stated it nearly in the same terms that he does, until ancient authority in medicine and its cognate sciences came to be despised, when it was entirely overlooked, until, as we have already mentioned, it was revived by Sir C. Bell.'

"As the writings of Galen are too voluminous for easy reference, and too expensive to be generally accessible, the following sketch of his more prominent views on the subject of the nervous system may not be unacceptable to the reader.

"'The nervous system consists of the brain, the spinal marrow, and the nerves.

"'The brain, including the cerebrum and cerebellum, is the immediate seat of the mind, and, as such, the primary organ of sensation and motion.

"'The brain is composed of the same substance as the nerves; the anterior portion is the softer, and gives origin to the nerves of sense; the posterior is harder, and gives origin to nerves of motion.

"'The spinal marrow is a production from the cerebellum, which however it exceeds in consistence. It contains just so much nervous matter as is necessary to form about sixty pairs of nerves, which are distributed to each part according to its demands for nervous energy.

"'Nerves have three uses: to communicate to the organs of sense their respective sentient faculties; to excite motion in the organs of motion; and to enable the organs of the body in general to discern what might be injurious to them. (*De Usu Part.* lib. v. c. 9.)

"'The nerves of the senses are soft, like the part of the brain from which they are derived: they all rise from the anterior part, and pursue a straight course to the organs which they supply.

"'The motory nerves are hard, arising from the posterior part of the brain, and the whole of the spinal marrow: these pursue a circuitous course to the parts to which they are distributed.'

"Although Galen thus recognised a distinction

between the sensatory and motory nerves, he conceived that this difference of function arose merely from difference of consistence. His idea appears to have been a mechanical one,—that the soft nerves were more susceptible of impressions, and the hard nerves less impressible, but stronger, and therefore better fitted for action. He had not the smallest notion of any original difference in the nature of the nervous power communicated by the two classes of nerves, nor that the parts of the central mass from which they spring were respectively the depositories of a sensific and a motific principle, distinct in their nature, and dependent on different modifications of the vital power. That he was entirely ignorant of all this, is evident from his maintaining that 'the hard motory nerves, although comparatively insusceptible of sensation, do nevertheless possess that faculty in a subordinate degree, and sufficiently to produce the general sense of touch;' and also that 'a nerve which originates as one of sensation from the soft part of the brain, may, at the same part of its course, become condensed in its texture, and assume the office of a motory nerve.' (*De Usu Part.* c. XIV.)

"The reader will perceive how little reason there is for Mr. Adams's assertion, that Galen anticipated Sir C. Bell's discovery of the sensatory and motory nerves, which consisted not in suggesting the probability that some nerves were distinct for sensation, and others for motion, but in showing, with reference to the spinal cord, that the anterior columns have exclusively the power of communicating motion, and the posterior that of receiving the impressions of sense. The diversity of function in the sensatory and motory nerves was ascribed by Galen to difference of texture, by Bell to difference of vital property; and with regard to the respective origin of these two classes of nerves, Galen *conjectured*, and was wrong, Bell *demonstrated*, and was right."

"It must be confessed," says Dr. Fletcher,* "that the ancients do not any of them appear to have been aware that this functional difference depended at all upon the different origin of the several nerves, conceiving that any branch of a nerve which was firm would convey volition, and any which was soft, would convey sensation in virtue of its texture alone. Similar doctrines were inculcated by Aretæus (*De Paralysi*), Rufus (*De Appel. Part.*) and other ancient authors, and more recently by Fallopius (*Obs. Anat.*), Willis (*Anat. Cereb.*), Van Swieten, Tissot, Cabanis, and numerous other writers; but the subject of the plurality of the nervous system had nevertheless been almost lost sight of [*in the modern sense, it cannot, as has been shown, be said to have ever been even hinted at*] in books, as well as in schools of anatomy and physiology, till it was revived (!) and presented to the world in a more or less collective form, and with many additions, by GALL, WALKER, BELLINGERI, BELL, MAGENDIE, MAYO,

* Rudiments of Physiology, pp. 91 and 92.

Earle, Arnold, and other contemporary authors, to whom we are indebted for almost all that has been established—if indeed any thing can be said to have been fully established—on the subject."

In the preceding paragraph, Dr. Fletcher, in chronological order, enumerates the modern writers on that which he denominates the plurality of the nervous system.

Gall, however, the first in order, contributed nothing to the great doctrine of our times: his plurality was of a very different, and altogether fantastic nature. "The most extravagant departure," says Sir C. Bell, "from all the legitimate modes of reasoning, although still under the colour of anatomical investigation, is the system of Dr. Gall. It is sufficient to say, that, without comprehending the grand divisions of the nervous system, without a notion of the distinct properties of the individual nerves, or having made any distinction of the columns of the spinal marrow, without even having ascertained the difference of cerebrum and cerebellum, Gall proceeded to describe the brain as composed of many particular and independent organs, and to assign to each the residence of some special faculty."

As to all the rest, Dr. Fletcher makes the following distinction, which, as marking the Two Parties, without any comment on either, may be useful to the reader.

"Mr. Walker," he says,* "regards the anterior roots of the spinal nerves as sensiferous, and the

* Rudiments of Physiology, p. 92.

posterior as motiferous, ministering at once to involuntary motion, by means of the filaments derived from the lateral or olivary columns, and to voluntary motion, by means of those derived from the proper posterior or cerebellic columns. On the other hand, SIR CHARLES BELL, MAYO, EARLE, ARNOLD, &c. inverting, as Mr. Walker says, *his* doctrine, represent the former as motiferous, and the latter as sensiferous."

THE CHIEF REMAINING QUESTION BETWEEN THESE TWO PARTIES WILL BE DECIDED WHENEVER IT IS DETERMINED—WHETHER MOTION, WHICH IS NATURAL AND NOT RETROGRADE, MUST ALWAYS HAVE ITS WHOLE APPROPRIATE COURSE, — OR, IN OTHER WORDS, WHETHER MOTION COMMUNICATED THROUGH DESCENDING MOTORY NERVES, MUST, WHEN NOT RETROGRADE, BE ALWAYS PRECEDED BY SENSATION OR IRRITATION EXCITED THROUGH ASCENDING SENSATORY NERVES, — AND WHETHER, WHEN NOT SO PRECEDED, IT IS NOT ALWAYS FORCED AND RETROGRADE ACTION.

To Mr. Walker's Papers, then, we first proceed; as, whether they be right or wrong as to function—direction or course, they are certainly those of by far the earliest writer who speaks of *nerves, spinal columns, and cerebral masses of sensation,—of the continuation of the action thence originating through the cerebrum,—and of other cerebral masses, spinal columns, and nerves of volition,—thus forming the great circle of nervous action and influence.*—This appears to be at least the first part of the discovery, "the conception or idea," as described by Professor Whewell.*

* "Confining myself to the discovery of the distinction of sensitive and motive nerves, I must remark that, according to the mode in which I have viewed all such events, the discovery consisted of two parts: the conception or idea, and the confirmation of this by facts.—*Letter to the Editor of the Medical Gazette.*

DOCUMENTS AND DATES

OF

DISCOVERY

IN THE

NERVOUS SYSTEM.

THOSE RELATIVE TO THE NERVOUS SYSTEM GENERALLY.

FUNCTION OF THE CEREBELLUM ASSIGNED;

BY ALEXANDER WALKER.

Date of Publication—1808.

This date is authenticated by three different publications— "*Tables of a Natural System of Medical Science,*" *having the date of* 1, *March,* 1808; "*Outline of a Natural System of Medical Science,*" *having the date of* 27, *October,* 1808; *and* "*Archives of Universal Science,*" *having the date of* 1, *January,* 1809.

The assignment of function constitutes the last column in each of the three sections of the following Table, which is inserted in all these works.

NATURAL ARRANGEMENT OF ORGANS.

Class I. Mechanical Organs.			Class II. Vital Organs.			Class III. Intellectual Organs.		
Order I. Bones, or Organs of Support.	*Order* II. Ligaments, or Organs of Connection.	*Order* III. Muscles, or Organs of Motion.	*Order* I. Lymphatics, &c. or Organs of Absorption.	*Order* II. Arteries, &c. or Organs of Circulation.	*Order* III. Glands, &c. or Organs of Secretion.	*Order* I. Eye, Ear, &c. or Organs of Sensation.	*Order* II. Cerebrum, or Organ of Perception, &c.	*Order* III. Cerebellum, &c. or Organ of Volition.

NATURAL ARRANGEMENT OF FUNCTIONS.

Class I. Mechanical Functions.			Class II. Vital Functions.			Class III. Intellectual Functions.		
Order I. Function of Support.	*Order* II. Function of Connection.	*Order* III. Function of Motion.	*Order* I. Function of Absorption.	*Order* II. Function of Circulation.	*Order* III. Function of Secretion.	*Order* I. Function of Sensation.	*Order* II. Function of Perception, &c.	*Order* III. Function of Volition.

NATURAL ARRANGEMENT OF DISEASES.

Class I. Diseases of the Mechanical Functions.			Class II. Diseases of the Vital Functions.			Class III. Diseases of the Intellectual Functions.		
Order I. Diseases of Support.	*Order* II. Diseases of Connection.	*Order* III. Diseases of Motion.	*Order* I. Diseases of Absorption.	*Order* II. Diseases of Circulation.	*Order* III. Diseases of Secretion.	*Order* I. Diseases of Sensation.	*Order* II. Diseases of Perception, &c.	*Order* III. Diseases of Volition.

N.B. The Genera under each order consist of Diminished, Disordered and Encreased Function; and the articles of Materia Medica hold an order precisely the reverse of the latter.

In a comparatively recent work, by the same physiologist, entitled "The Nervous System, Anatomical and Physiological: in which the functions of the various parts of the brain are for the first time assigned; and to which is prefixed some account of the author's earliest discoveries, of which the more recent doctrine of Bell, Magendie, etc. is shown to be at once a plagiarism, an inversion, and a blunder, associated with useless experiments, which they have neither understood nor explained," the author gives the following brief history of this assignment.

"To the distinction of the nerves, as forming two classes, namely those of sensation and those of volition, the writer was, in some measure, led by the fundamental fact just now stated, as to the cerebel; for he could not see in it an organ of volition, without concluding that the nervous cords connecting it with the muscles belonged to the same function, and must be totally distinct from those which connect the organs of sense with the cerebrum or greater brain, and which therefore transmit sensations.

"In 'Tables of a Natural System of Medical Science,' proposed by the writer, and printed by Messrs. Oliver and Boyd, of Edinburgh, on the 1st of March, 1808, as appears from the tables themselves, he first, in a printed work, assigned the function of will or volition to the cerebel; though he had held, and occasionally taught that doctrine ever since the year 1803.

"In 'Outline of a Natural System of Medical

Science,' forming his preliminary lectures, dedicated to Dr. Monro, sen., printed at the university press, on the 27th of October, of the same year, and published by Sir R. Phillips, in London, and by Bryce and Co., at Edinburgh, the same use was, in an accompanying table, assigned to that organ.

"In 'Archives of Universal Science,' vol. i. for January, 1809, published at Edinburgh on the first of that month, this was repeated.—Thus, for the third time within the year 1808, was this function assigned by the writer; for, even as to the last work, it will be allowed, that a volume of nearly 400 pages, published on the first day of 1809, must have been sent to press and printed in 1808.

"At this time, the writer had not attained his subsequent ideas of the nervous system: he imagined the nerves to be more especially dependent upon or associated with the cerebel in the function of will, or volition; and he treated them as such, both in these works and in his unpublished lectures.

"In the second volume of the work last quoted, for April, 1809, the writer, now associating the spinal cord with the cerebel in the production of volition, and considering certain nerves (for he now divided them into two kinds, nerves of sensation and nerves of volition) as merely the means of transmitting voluntary impulses—expressed himself," as in that and subsequent Papers, here inserted.

EXTRACTS FROM

GENERAL PHYSIOLOGY OF THE INTELLECTUAL ORGANS.

BY ALEXANDER WALKER.

Date of Publication — April, 1809.

This paper is extracted from "Archives of Universal Science," Volume II, for April, 1809, *page* 167, *et seq.*

GENERAL ARRANGEMENT OF THE INTELLECTUAL ORGANS.—The kinds of Intellectual Organs are five in number; and, if ARRANGED IN THE ORDER OF THE DEPENDENCE OF THEIR FUNCTIONS, THEY STAND THUS; ORGANS OF SENSE, NERVES OF SENSATION, CEREBRUM, CEREBELLUM AND SPINAL MARROW, AND NERVES OF VOLITION.

By mind, I mean merely the functions of the intellectual organs, namely sensation, mental operation and volition, which evidently are to the organs of sense, brain and nerves, precisely what absorption, circulation and secretion are to the lymphatics, blood-vessels and glands, or what support, connection and motion are to the bones, ligaments and muscles; nor is there any thing more mysterious in the first of these series of functions than in the last of them. It is indeed strange that sensation, mental operation and volition should ever have been thought less implicitly dependent upon the organs of sense, brain and nerves than all the other functions of the body are upon their respective organs.

FUNCTION OF THE ORGANS OF SENSE, OR OF SENSATION.—So close is the analogy in the functions of all the organs of sense, that tasting, smelling, seeing and hearing seem merely to be different modifications of touch.

That all sensation is a mere modification of touch is proved by comparative as well as by human anatomy; for the horns of the snail and the whole superficies of many animals are at once their organ of touch, taste, smell, seeing and hearing; or, in other words, are susceptible of impressions from all those forms and actions of matter which, in the more perfect animals, impress distinct organs.

That sensation belongs entirely to the organs of sense, is clearly proven by this, that several animals possessing a brain retain sensation (in this case improperly termed irritability) unimpaired long after it is removed.

Muscular irritability, when a nerve is tied or cut, is a beautiful specimen of sensation existing without perception. But the intestines, in their peristaltic motion, afford a similar specimen even in the healthy state.

Nor is this opinion, in the slightest degree, invalidated by patients falsely seeming to have sensation even in amputated extremities; because, in such cases, the sensation, if it can be said to exist (though it may properly be termed a deception or mistake), exists merely at the extreme surface of the remaining portion. "The pain or sensation," says Dr. Darwin, "which formerly had arisen in the foot or toes, and been propagated along the nerves to the central part of the sensorium, was at the same time accompanied with a visible idea of the shape and place, and with a tangible idea of the solidity of the affected limb: now when these nerves are afterwards affected by an injury done to the remaining stump, with a similar degree or kind of pain, the ideas of the shape, place, or solidity of the lost limb, return *by association;* as these ideas belong to the organs of sight and touch, on which they were first excited."

The whole of *the common error upon this subject, arises from not distinguishing between sensation and perception; the latter of which can exist only in a sensorium commune,* and is, in its nature, somewhat different from the former.

The truth of this remark unavoidably destroys that supposed unity of mind which was inconsistent with all the phenomena of the intellectual functions.

All the other intellectual functions are nevertheless modifications of sensation.

Soemmering has observed, that man has the

largest brain in proportion to the nerves given off from it, and that this proportional magnitude may, in every instance, be referred to as the best criterion of the degrees of intelligence. Now it appears to me not at all difficult to account for this fact (the general truth of which may be granted) by comparing it with another not less important, viz. that, in the inferior classes of animals, the nervous system becomes, as we descend, more and more widely diffused.

Now the more equally distributed this system is, the more independent of each other are the parts of organised beings.

Animals having this sensitive substance very generally diffused, when mutilated, recover their figure, or when cut into pieces, form several individuals, having each a system of sensation and volition. Animals having this system perhaps generally diffused, as the polyp, having been divided into the smallest fragments, each fragment self exists, and becomes a perfect individual.

Yet these polyps, thus minutely divisible and destitute of perception, have great sensibility. Their sense of touch is exquisite, and they not only feel the slightest motion of water, but all the degrees of heat and light. To the last of these the hydra is very sensible, as it always turns to it, and seems to enjoy it. The Actiniæ also expand in exact correspondence to the serenity of the atmosphere.

The sensibility of these animals [some worms] is

so limited in extent, that if a thread dipt in a solution of salt be thrown across their bodies, a stricture will take place merely under the thread; it never extends to the excitement of a perception throughout the animal.

FUNCTION OF THE NERVES OF SENSATION.—The division of nerves into those of motion and those of sensation is absurd, because all nerves are nerves of motion; THE PROPER DIVISION IS INTO NERVES OF SENSATION AND NERVES OF VOLITION, OR NERVES OF IMPRESSION AND NERVES OF EXPRESSION.

Now as, in some cases, sensation exists without volition, and as almost all nerves arise by distinct filaments, I am of opinion, that wherever a part, having both sensation and motion, is supplied from one nervous trunk, that trunk envelopes both a nerve of sensation and one of volition.

The nerves, it is known, are the sole means of action, and it appears to me that different sensations are conveyed by them, in consequence of different motions being excited in them by different external objects.

That the nervous matter is so gross as to be affected by pressure is evident from this, that the compression of a nerve excites a muscle to act; and it is indeed also proved by actual demonstration. It does not even appear, that great subtilty is necessary in these motions of the nervous substance.

"When the idea of solidity is excited," says Dr.

Darwin, "a part of the extensive organ of touch is compressed by some external body, and this part of the sensorium, so compressed, exactly resembles *in figure* the figure of the body that compresses it. Hence, when we acquire the idea of solidity, we acquire, at the same time the idea of *figure;* and this idea of figure, or motion of *a part* of the organ of touch, exactly resembles *in its figure* the figure of the body that occasions it ; and thus exactly acquaints us with this of the external world."

FUNCTIONS OF THE CEREBRUM. — To sensation, which is the function of the organs of sense, succeeds, in the more perfect animals, perception, which is the function of the brain, or more properly of the cerebrum.

Now *as we have shown, that sensation is implicitly dependent upon motion, and as this and all the other functions of the brain are entirely the results or modifications of sensation, they also must be dependent on motion.* And this is confirmed by the medullary substance of the brain consisting entirely of fine fibres in various directions, seemingly for the purpose of communicating motion like the nerves, and, by the slightest change of structure, uniformly causing a corresponding change of action, and consequently of mental operation.

We know, that all operations are the result of motion, and as we also know, that motion never terminates in one body without being communicated to contiguous ones, therefore, even in the most secret of all operations, there must exist a series of motions, the infallible property of which is, from a cause to produce effects by bringing bodies either into connection by media or into actual contact.

The argument, therefore, which Mr. Hume, in support of his peculiar doctrine, borrows from anatomy, namely, that the power by which muscular motion is performed is mysterious and unintelligible, and that effects of which we are ignorant, and in themselves totally different from those intended, are first produced—this argument, I say, is false; because the effect produced differs from that intended, only in as much as the termination of motion differs from its commencement. For *the beautiful perpetuation of the same species of motion in the vital actions, is at once an excellent illustration, and an analogical proof of similarly continued motion in the intellectual functions.*

The same argument applied by Mr. Hume to prove, that we are conscious of no power in the mind, when by an act or command of the will, we raise up a new idea, fix the mind to the contemplation of it, turn it on all sides, and, at last, dismiss it for some other idea, when we think that we have surveyed it with sufficient accuracy, is equally refuted by the same observation, and must appear strikingly false, when, in addition to this, it is observed, that all his terms '*act* or *command* of the will,' '*raise up* an idea;' '*fix* the mind;' '*turn* the idea on all sides;' '*dismiss* the idea,' express nothing but motion and consequently power, and at once refute his assertion.

Mr. Locke, indeed, in his work on the human understanding, says, "As to the manner in which bodies produce ideas in us; it is manifestly by impulse, the only way which we can conceive bodies to operate in."

Dr. Darwin, in his Zoonomia, says, "The word *idea* has various meanings in the writers of metaphysics: it is here used simply for those notions of external things, which our organs of sense bring us acquainted with originally; and is defined a *contraction*, or *motion*, or *configuration*, of the fibres, which constitute the immediate organ of sense. Synonymous with the word idea, we shall sometimes use the words sensual motion in contradistinction to muscular motion;" and, in another place, he says, "In some convulsive diseases, a delirium or insanity supervenes, and the convulsions cease; and conversely the convulsions shall supervene, and the delirium cease. Of this I have been a witness many times in a day in the paroxysms of violent epilepsies; which evinces that one kind of delirium is a convulsion of the organs of sense, and that our ideas are the *motions* of these organs."

As all language, therefore, relative to the mind, expresses motion, and as we cannot even have an idea of its operations without motion, any denial of this must consequently have its foundation, since not in reason, certainly in prejudice.

Thus evident motion takes place in impression, a less evident, but still acknowledged one, in mental operation, and again, an evident one in the acts of volition. But motion not only demonstrates itself in impression; seems continued in judging; and again, evidences itself in expression; but beautifully corresponding to the general laws of the most evident species of motion, it does not terminate here without communicating new and similar motions — another series of impressions, ideas, emotions, passions and volitions, to other minds.

If to all this it be objected, that matter and motion cannot produce these wonderful effects, I have only to observe, that the combinations of matter in its grossest forms, viz. the mixture of the seminal and ovarian fluids, actually produces the organs of sense, brain and nerves — the intellectual organs of the whole race of animals; and that as the actions of all bodies depend upon their structure, consequently the actions or the functions of these parts have the same origin. All vegetables also depend for their existence on an analogous secretion.

To perception succeed the more complex operations of mind, which consciousness accompanies in all their stages, and memory or imagination recall when they have passed.

FUNCTION OF THE CEREBELLUM AND MEDULLA SPINALIS, OR VOLITION.—*The cerebellum and medulla spinalis appear to me, from numerous observations, to be the organ of volition.*

The inferior animals, however defective in intellect, possess motion; and in almost all of them that have any visible nervous system a cerebellum—its organ, exists.

As sensation and volition seem exactly opposed to each other, so is the face, containing the organs of sense, to the cavity containing the cerebellum. The analogy also attends their situation in all animals; for as, in the inferior classes, the face advances, the cerebellum uniformly recedes, and both are generally separated from the cerebrum either by membranes, or by bony plates.

Man also has the greatest cerebrum, compared with his cerebellum, and has likewise most of intellect, though not most of locomotion.

FUNCTION OF THE NERVES OF VOLITION. — *The only apparent difference between the nerves of sensation and those of volition, is, that their motions take place in different directions.*—THE LATTER, THEREFORE, MAY BE SAID TO RESEMBLE THE ARTERIES; THE FORMER THE VEINS.

It is certain, however, that motion exists to great excess without perception. The gadfly has the most rapid motions, but seems scarcely to possess perception.

That the irritation, however, of either muscles or nerves when separated, produces contraction, either proves that motion in these nerves, occasionally takes place in both directions, or that the two kinds of nerves are connected at various points throughout their course, and that the influence of a single impulse is thus permitted to extend in every direction. At all events it proves, that the functions of nerves remain some time, though cut off from the brain, and that perception is not necessary to precede expression.*

* Irritability is a compound term, at once expressing sensibility and evident motion.

EXTRACTS FROM

"NEW ANATOMY AND PHYSIOLOGY OF THE BRAIN IN PARTICULAR, AND OF THE NERVOUS SYSTEM IN GENERAL."

BY ALEXANDER WALKER.

Date of Publication — July, 1809.

This paper is extracted from "Archives of Universal Science," Volume III, for July, 1809, *page* 172, *et seq.*

I HAVE entitled this paper, "New Anatomy and Physiology of the Brain," &c., because, while the whole of the physiology which it delivers is original, all the leading facts of anatomy upon which that physiology is founded, such as the general course of the medullary matter, the double origins, as they are termed, of the nerves, &c. are not less so. The object of this paper consequently prevents my entering into such details as are known to every one, and limits me to the notice of such facts as are either entirely original, or, from being placed in a new point of view, admit of original conclusions. The paper is, therefore, a brief one, though, from the magnitude of the anatomical facts and physiological reasonings which it delivers, it presents a connected system both of the anatomy and physiology of the nervous system in general, and of the brain in particular.

ANATOMY.

Although the face and cerebellum are, in different animals, very differently placed with regard to the cerebrum, yet there is a peculiar relation between the situation of one of these and that of the other, with regard to it. In other words, although the face is sometimes in one situation and sometimes in another with relation to the cerebrum, yet to each given variation of its situation with regard to that body, there is a corresponding and uniformly accompanying variation in the situation of the cerebellum. Thus, in man, as the face is placed below the anterior part of the cerebrum, so the cerebellum is placed below its posterior part, and precisely as in the inferior animals the face advances, precisely so does the cerebellum recede, till, in those animals in which the face is placed exactly before it, the cerebellum is placed exactly behind it. Moreover, both the face and cerebellum are in general separated from the cerebrum either by membranes or by bony plates. Thus, an analogy always exists with regard to their situation.

Both of these masses are, generally speaking, composed of two substances—a medullary and a cineritious. I shall especially treat of the arrangement of the first, in the following paragraphs:

THE MEDULLARY MATTER MAY BE TRACED AS CONTINUED FROM THE PORTIONS OF MANY NERVES WHICH JOIN THE TWO ANTERIOR COLUMNS OF THE SPINAL MARROW, UPWARD THROUGH THESE COLUMNS TO THE INFERIOR FASCICULI OF THE MEDULLA OBLONGATA, FORWARD THROUGH THE CRURA CEREBRI, AND FORWARD, OUTWARD AND UPWARD THROUGH THE CORPORA STRIATA, AND THE HEMISPHERES OF THE CEREBRUM.

FROM THE HEMISPHERES IT PASSES POSTERIORLY, BACKWARD, INWARD AND DOWNWARD THROUGH THE THALAMI, BACKWARD THROUGH THE STRIÆ INFERIOR TO THE NATES AND TESTES, AND BACKWARD AND UPWARD THROUGH THE PROCESSUS CEREBELLI AD TESTES, OR THE ANTERIOR PEDUNCLES OF THE CEREBELLUM, TO THE SUBSTANCE OF THE CEREBELLUM ITSELF.*

* In making a section of the thalamus, the divided striæ appear most numerous toward its upper and outer, and much more scattered towards its inner side; and in dividing still downward, a section of the crus cerebri appears inferiorly. By making a second section about the middle of the thalamus, its exterior superior filaments appear to unite into a denser semicircular form, the convexity of which is still toward its outer and upper side, and, at the lower part of which, the crus cerebri appears still more distinct. By making a third section, this arrangement becomes still more evident, but, at the same time more contracted, and passes more toward the inner and under side of the Nates and Testis, gradually approaching the processus cerebelli ad testem or the anterior peduncle of the cerebellum. A horizontal incision also, if made immediately below the

LASTLY, FROM THE CEREBELLUM, IT PASSES DOWNWARD BY THE CORPORA RESTIFORMIA, SUPERIOR FASCICULI OF THE MEDULLA, PROCESSUS CEREBELLI AD MEDULLAM OR POSTERIOR PEDUNCLES OF THE CEREBELLUM, TO THE POSTERIOR COLUMNS OF THE SPINAL MARROW, AND THE REMAINING PORTIONS OF THE NUMEROUS NERVES WHICH JOIN IT.

THUS THE MEDULLARY FIBRES FORM A MOST REMARKABLE CIRCLE, OF WHICH THIS IS THE DIRECT COURSE.*

PHYSIOLOGY.

From the peculiar opposition which subsists between the situation of the face and cerebellum, we are entitled to expect a similar opposition in their functions. As the face, therefore, occupied by the chief organs of sense, is the seat of sensation, so we might expect the cerebellum to be the organ of volition. This supposition receives additional force

level of this semicircular tract, shows that the striæ of the thalami terminate in a longitudinal fasciculus, which passing inferiorly and interiorly to the natis and testis, terminates in this peduncle. Thus are the cerebrum and cerebellum connected by the medullary substance.

* In many sections of the cerebrum and cerebellum, these directions of the medullary filaments are very apparent. In making a vertical section of the cerebellum, its ascending and descending filaments become frequently very evident; they seem to differ, by a slight shading, in colour, owing doubtless to the different arrangement of their particles; and they appear to bend slightly around each other.

from the consideration that, as the organs of sense and the cerebellum are the first and the last portions of the nervous system, so sensation and volition are the first and the last of its functions. But this supposition is completely confirmed, when we recollect, that the degrees of voluntary power always bear a close analogy to the various magnitudes of the cerebellum. In fishes, for instance, which possess amazing locomotive power, the cerebellum is often larger than the hemispheres!

THE COURSE OF THE ACTIONS IN THE OTHER MATTER—THE MEDULLARY, IS PRECISELY THE SAME WITH THAT OF THE STRUCTURE ITSELF, AS I HAVE DESCRIBED IT. For, it is evident, that two species of action take place through this structure—one obviously advancing from the organs of sense toward the sensorium commune, and another returning from the sensorium commune to actuate the muscles and produce locomotion. Now, it does not accord with the distinctness of natural operations to suppose, that these motions in opposite directions take place through one and the same series of particles. It is far more accordant with that distinctness, to suppose, that they take place through different series. And this becomes confirmed when we observe that circuitous course of the medullary fibres of the brain which in this paper I have described, the double columns of the spinal marrow, which have for some time been known, but have never hitherto been traced in connection with that general course, and the double origins, as they are termed, even of the encephalic nerves, which I have here pointed out. Nature, thus, presents to us the double means by which this double operation is effected.

But it may be questioned by which nerves, columns and cerebral masses, the action ascends to the brain, and by which it descends to the muscles. Fortunately, here nature also directs us. Several nerves of mere sensation join the anterior masses; hence, they must be the ascending: one nerve of mere locomotion proceeds from the posterior masses; hence, they must be the descending—for sensation, as already said, must ascend to, and volition must descend from the sensorium commune.

Thus, then, it is proved to us, that *medullary action commences in the organs of sense; passes, in a general manner, to the spinal marrow, by the anterior fasciculi of the spinal nerves, which are, therefore, nerves of sensation, and the connexions of which with the spinal marrow or brain must be termed their spinal or cerebral* TERMINATIONS; *ascends through the anterior columns of the spinal marrow which are, therefore, its ascending columns; passes forward through the inferior fasciculi of the medulla oblongata, and then through the crura cerebri; extends forward, outward and upward through the corpora striata; and reaches the hemispheres of the cerebrum itself. This precisely is the course of its ascent to the sensorium commune.*

From the posterior part of the medulla of the hemispheres, it returns by the thalami, passing backward, inward and downward; flows backward in the fasciculi under the nates and testes; backward and upward through the processus cerebelli ad testes or anterior peduncles of the cerebellum; and thus reaches the medulla of the cerebellum itself.

From the cerebellum, it descends through the posterior columns of the spinal marrow, which are, therefore, its descending columns; and expands through the posterior fasciculi of all the nerves, which are, therefore, the nerves of volition, and the connexions of which with the spinal marrow or brain must be termed their spinal or cerebellic ORIGINS. *This precisely is the course of its descent from the sensorium commune toward the muscular system.*

Now, from this course, it is evident, that impressions acting on the organs of sense, and there producing sensations, will reach, by this route, the sensorium commune, and there constitute perception, or, in other words, will have their influence diffused from this central point, and rendered universally cognizable to the system; for all the actions which take place in this system must be cognizable to it, and even the action of other systems can only be cognizable by means of this one.

Volition would similarly appear to consist in the transmission of the impulse from the cerebellum, the new modification which, from its structure, that impulse must undergo, and its rapid descent through the posterior columns to the muscular organs.

IDEA OF A NEW ANATOMY OF THE BRAIN;

SUBMITTED FOR THE OBSERVATIONS OF HIS FRIENDS;

BY CHARLES BELL, F.R.S.E.

Date of Printing (the work was never published) — 1811.

It is not a little curious that Mr. Shaw, a friend and relative of Sir C. Bell, in the Medico-Chirurgical Transactions, Vol. XII, Part I, page 149, *should expressly have said, " Sir C. Bell's short essay on the Anatomy of the Brain was printed in* 1809;" *and, as M. Magendie's Second Paper—"Expériences sur les Fonctions des Racines des Nerfs qui naissent de la Moëlle Epinière," was published in* 1822, *and Mr. Shaw then claimed a precedence of thirteen years for Sir C. Bell, it is evident that Mr. Shaw again ascribed to this pamphlet the date of* 1809!!!

This date was repeated in Papers, Reviews, Pamphlets, &c.; yet Sir C. Bell did not think it necessary, for many years, to correct this error.

In his work, however, entitled " The Nervous System," published in 1830, *Sir C. Bell, at last, formally and repeatedly abandoned all claim to that date. In page* 14, *he says,—" I printed a little work in* 1811, *which I entitled ' An Idea of a New Anatomy of the Brain, submitted for the observation of the Author's Friends.' " And again, page* 21, *he says,—" The ' Idea of a New Anatomy of the Brain, &c.' was published [printed, it should be] in* 1811."

TO PREVENT THE POSSIBILITY OF THIS PAPER BEING SUPPOSED TO CONTAIN WHAT IT DOES NOT CONTAIN, IT IS HERE GIVEN ENTIRE; AND ITS NEAREST APPROACHES TO THE NEW DOCTRINES ARE PRINTED IN ITALICS OR SMALL CAPITALS.—SIR C. BELL DOES NOT PRETEND TO HAVE MADE ANY FURTHER ADVANCE TILL 1821,—TEN YEARS AFTER THIS.

NOTE.

The want of any consistent history of the Brain and Nerves, and the dull unmeaning manner which is in use of demonstrating the brain, may authorize any novelty in the manner of treating the subject.

I have found some of my friends so mistaken in their conceptions of the object of the demonstrations which I have delivered in my lectures, that I wish to vindicate myself at all hazards. They would have it that I am in search of the seat of the soul; but I wish only to investigate the structure of the brain, as we examine the structure of the eye and ear.

It is not more presumptuous to follow the tracts of nervous matter in the brain, and to attempt to discover the course of sensation, than it is to trace the rays of light through the humours of the eye, and to say, that the retina is the seat of vision. Why are we to close the investigation with the discovery of the external organ?

It would have been easy to have given this Essay an imposing splendour, by illustrations and engravings of the parts, but I submit it as a sketch to those who are well able to judge of it *in this shape.*

The prevailing doctrine of the anatomical schools is, that the whole brain is a common sensorium; that the extremities of the nerves are organized, so that each is fitted to receive a peculiar impression; or that they are distinguished from each other only by delicacy of structure, and by a corresponding delicacy of sensation; that the nerve of the eye, for example, differs from the nerves of touch only in the degree of its sensibility.

It is imagined that impressions, thus differing in kind, are carried along the nerves to the sensorium, and presented to the mind; and that the mind, by the same nerves which receive sensation, sends out the mandate of the will to the moving parts of the body.

It is further imagined, that there is a set of nerves, called vital nerves, which are less strictly connected with the sensorium, or which have upon them knots, cutting off the course of sensation, and thereby excluding the vital motions from the government of the will.

This appears sufficiently simple and consistent, until we begin to examine anatomically the structure of the brain, and the course of the nerves, — then all is confusion: the divisions and subdivisions of the brain, the circuitous course of nerves, their intricate connections, their separation and re-union, are puzzling in the last degree, and are indeed considered as things inscrutable. Thus it is that he who knows the parts the best, is most in a maze, and he who knows least of anatomy, sees least inconsistency in the commonly received opinion.

In opposition to these opinions, I have to offer reasons for believing that *the cerebrum and cerebellum are different in function as in form;* that the parts of the cerebrum have different functions; and that the nerves which we trace in the body are not single nerves possessing various powers, but bundles of different nerves, whose filaments are united for the convenience of distribution, but which are distinct in office, as they are in origin from the brain.

That the external organs of the senses have the matter of the nerves adapted to receive certain impressions, while the corresponding organs of the brain are put in activity by the external excitement: That the idea or perception is according to the part of the brain to which the nerve is attached, and that each organ has a certain limited number of changes to be wrought upon it by the external impression.

That *the nerves of sense, the nerves of motion, and the vital nerves, are distinct through their whole course, though they seem sometimes united in one bundle*; and that they depend for their attributes on the organs of the brain to which they are severally attached.

The view which I have to present will serve to shew why there are divisions, and many distinct parts in the brain; why some nerves are simple in their origin and distribution, and others intricate beyond description. It will explain the apparently accidental connection between the twigs of nerves. It will do away the difficulty of conceiving how sensation and volition should be the operation of the same nerve at the same moment. It will shew how a nerve may lose one property and retain another; and it will give an interest to the labours of the anatomist in tracing the nerves.

IDEA, &c.

WHEN in contemplating the structure of the eye we say, how admirably it is adapted to the laws of light! we use language which implies a partial, and consequently an erroneous view. And the philosopher takes not a more enlarged survey of Nature when he declares how curiously the laws of light are adapted to the constitution of the eye.

This Creation, of which we are a part, has not been formed in parts. The organ of vision, and the matter or influence carried to the organ, and the qualities of bodies with which we are acquainted through it, are parts of a system great beyond our imperfect comprehension, formed as it should seem at once in wisdom; not pieced together like the work of human ingenuity.

When this whole was created (of which the remote planetary system, as well as our bodies, and the objects more familiar to our observation, are but parts) the mind was placed in a body not merely suited to its residence, but in circumstances to be moved by the materials around it; and the capacities of the mind, and the powers of the organs, which are as a medium betwixt the mind and the external world, have an original constitution framed in relation to the qualities of things.

It is admitted that neither bodies nor the images of bodies enter the brain. It is indeed impossible to believe that colour can be conveyed along a nerve; or the vibration in which we suppose sound to consist can be retained in the brain: but we can conceive, and have reason to believe, that an impression is made upon the organs of the outward senses, when we see, or hear, or taste.

In this enquiry, it is most essential to observe, that while each organ of sense is provided with a capacity of receiving certain changes to be played upon it, as it were, yet each is utterly incapable of receiving the impression destined for another organ of sensation.

It is also very remarkable that an impression made on two different nerves of sense, though with the same instrument, will produce two distinct sensations; and the ideas resulting will only have relation to the organ affected.

As the announcing of these facts forms a natural introduction to the Anatomy of the Brain, which I am about to deliver, I shall state them more fully.

There are four kinds of Papillæ on the tongue, but with two of those only we have to do at present. Of these, the Papillæ of one kind form the seat of the sense of taste; the other Papillæ (more numerous and smaller) resemble the extremities of the nerves in the common skin, and are the organs of touch in the tongue. When I take a sharp steel point and touch one of *these* Papillæ, I feel the sharpness. The sense of *touch* informs me of the shape of the instrument. When I touch a Papilla of taste, I have sensation similar to the former. I know not that a point touches the tongue, but I am sensible of a metallic taste, and the sensation passes backward on the tongue.

In the operation of couching the cataract, the pain of piercing the retina with a needle is not so great as that which proceeds from a grain of sand under the eyelid. And although the derangement of the stomach sometimes marks the injury of an organ so delicate, yet the pain is occasioned by piercing the outward coat, not by the affection of the expanded nerve of vision.

If the sensation of light were conveyed to us by the retina, the organ of vision, in consequence of that organ being as much more sensible than the surface of the body as the impression of light is more delicate than that pressure which gives us the sense of touch; what would be the feelings of a man subjected to an operation in which a needle were pushed through the nerve? Life could not bear so great a pain.

But there is an occurrence during this operation on the eye, which will direct us to the truth: when the needle pierces the eye, the patient has the sensation of a spark of fire before the eye.

This fact is corroborated by experiments made on

the eye. When the eye-ball is pressed on the side, we perceive various coloured light. Indeed, the mere effect of a blow on the head might inform us, that sensation depends on the exercise of the organ affected, not on the impression conveyed to the external organ; for by the vibration caused by the blow, the ears ring, and the eye flashes light, while there is neither light nor sound present.

It may be said that there is here no proof of the sensation being in the brain more than in the external organ of sense. But when the nerve of a stump is touched, the pain is as if in the amputated extremity. If it be still said that this is no proper example of a peculiar sense existing without its external organ, I offer the following example: Quando penis glandem exedat ulcus, et nihil nisi granulatio maneat, ad extremam tamen nervi pudicæ pactem ubi terminatur sensus supersunt, et exquisitissima sensus gratificatio.

If light, pressure, galvanism, or electricity produce vision, we must conclude that the idea in the mind is the result of an action excited in the eye or in the brain, not of any thing received, though caused by an impression from without. The operations of the mind are confined, not by the limited nature of things created, but by the limited number of our organs of sense. By induction we know that things exist which yet are not brought under the operation of the senses. When we have never known the operation of one of the organs of the five senses, we can never know the ideas pertaining to that sense; and what would be the effect on our minds, even constituted as they now are, with a superadded organ of sense, no man can distinctly imagine.

As we are parts of the creation, so God has bound us to the material world, by this law of our nature, that it shall require excitement from without, and an operation produced by the action of things external to rouse our faculties: but that once brought into activity, the organs can be put in exercise by the mind, and be made to minister to the memory and the imagination, and all the faculties of the soul.

I shall hereafter show, that the operations of the mind are seated in the great mass of the cerebrum, while the parts of the brain to which the nerves of sense tend, strictly form the seat of the sensation, being the internal organs of sense. These organs are operated upon in two directions. They receive the impression from without, as from the eye and ear: and as their action influences the operations of the brain producing perception, so are they brought into action, and suffer changes similar to that which they experience from external pressure by the operation of the will; or, as I am now treating of the subject anatomically, by the operation of the great mass of the brain upon them.

In all regulated actions of the muscles, we must acknowledge that they are influenced through the same nerves, by the same operation of the sensorium. Now the operations of the body are as nice and curious, and as perfectly regulated before reason has sway, as they are at any time after, when the muscular frame might be supposed to be under the guidance of sense and reason. Instinctive motions are the operations of the same organs, the brain and nerves and muscles, which minister reason and volition in our mature years. When the young of any animal turns to the nipple, directed by the sense of smelling, the same operations are performed, and through the same means, as afterwards when we make an effort to avoid what is noxious, or desire and move towards what is agreeable.

The operations of the brain may be said to be threefold: 1. The frame of the body is endowed with the characters of life, and the vital parts held together as one system through the operation of the brain and nerves; and the secret operations of the vital organs suffer the controul of the brain, though we are unconscious of the thousand delicate operations which are every instant going on in the body. 2. In the second place, the instinctive motions which precede the development of the intellectual faculties are performed through the brain and nerves. 3. In the last place, the operation of the senses in rousing the faculties of the mind, and the exercise of the mind over the moving parts of the body, is through the brain and nerves. The first of these is perfect in nature and independent of the mind. The second is a prescribed and limited operation of the instrument of thought and agency. The last begins by imperceptible degrees, and has no limit in extent and variety. It is that to which all the rest is subservient, the end being the calling into activity and the sustaining of an intellectual being.

Thus we see that in as far as is necessary to the great system, the operation of the brain, nerves, and muscles are perfect from the beginning; and we are naturally moved to ask, might not the operations of the mind have been thus perfect and spontaneous from the beginning as well as slowly excited into action by outward impressions? Then man would have been an insulated being, not only cut off from the inanimate world around him, but from his fellows; he would have been an individual, not a part of a whole. That he may have a motive and a spring to action, and suffer pain and pleasure, and become an intelligent being, answerable for his actions,—sensation is made to result from external impression, and reason and passion to come from the experience of good and evil; first, as they are in reference to his corporeal frame, and finally, as they belong to the intellectual privations and enjoyments.

The brain is a mass of soft matter, in part of a white colour, and generally striated; in part of a grey or cineritious colour, having no fibrous appearance. It has grand divisions and subdivisions: and as the forms exist before the solid bone encloses the brain; and as the distinctions of parts are equally observable in animals whose brain is surrounded with fluid, they evidently are not accidental, but are a consequence of internal structure; or, in other words, they have a correspondence with distinctions in the uses of the parts of the brain.

On examining the grand divisions of the brain, we are forced to admit that there are four brains. For the brain is divided longitudinally by a deep fissure; and the line of distinction can even be traced where the sides are united in substance. Whatever we observe on one side has a corresponding part on the other; and an exact resemblance and symmetry is preserved in all the lateral divisions of the brain. And so, if we take the proof of anatomy, we must admit that as the nerves are double, and the organs of sense double, so is the brain double; and every sensation conveyed to the brain is conveyed to the two lateral parts; and the operations performed must be done in both lateral portions at the same moment.

I speak of the lateral divisions of the brain being distinct brains combined in function, in order more strongly to mark the distinction betwixt the anterior and posterior grand divisions. Betwixt the lateral parts there is a strict resemblance in form and substance: each principal part is united by transverse tracts of medullary matter; and there is every provision for their acting with perfect sympathy. On the contrary, the *cerebrum*, the anterior grand division, and the *cerebellum*, the posterior grand division, have slight and indirect connection. In form and division of parts, and arrangement of white and grey matter, there is no resemblance. There is here nothing of that symmetry and correspondence of parts which is so remarkable betwixt the right and left portions.

I have found evidence that the vascular system of the cerebellum may be affected independently of the vessels of the cerebrum. I have seen the whole surface of the cerebellum studded with spots of extravasated blood as small as pin-heads, so as to be quite red, while no mark of disease was upon the surface of the cerebrum. The action of vessels, it is needless to say, is under the influence of the parts to which they go; and in this we have a proof of a distinct state of activity in the cerebrum and cerebellum.

From these facts, were there no other, we are entitled to conclude that in the operations excited in the brain there cannot be such sympathy or corresponding movement in the cerebrum and cerebellum as there is betwixt the lateral portions of the cerebrum; that the anterior and posterior grand divisions of the brain perform distinct offices.

In examining this subject further, we find, when we compare the relative magnitude of the cerebrum to the other parts of the brain in man and in brutes, that in the latter the cerebrum is much smaller, having nothing of the relative magnitude and importance which in man it bears to the other parts of the nervous system; signifying that the cerebrum is the seat of those qualities of mind which distinguish man. We may observe also that the posterior grand division, or cerebellum, remains more permanent in form: while the cerebrum changes in conformity to the organs of sense, or the endowments of the different classes of animals. In the inferior animals, for example, where there are two external organs of the same sense, there is to be found two distinct corresponding portions of cerebrum, while the cerebellum corresponds with the frame of the body.

In thinking of this subject, it is natural to expect that we should be able to put the matter to proof by experiment. But how is this to be accomplished, since any experiment direct upon the brain itself must be difficult, if not impossible?—I took this view of the subject. *The medulla spinalis has a central division, and also a distinction into anterior and posterior fasciculi, corresponding with the anterior and posterior portions of the brain. Further* WE CAN TRACE DOWN THE CRURA OF THE CEREBRUM INTO THE ANTERIOR FASCICULUS OF THE SPINAL MARROW, AND THE CRURA OF THE CEREBELLUM INTO THE POSTERIOR FASCICULUS. I thought that here I might have an opportunity of touching the *cerebellum*, as it were, through the posterior portion of the spinal marrow, and the *cerebrum* by the anterior portion. To this end, I made experiments which, though they were not conclusive, encouraged me in the view I had taken.

I found that injury done to the anterior portion of the spinal marrow, convulsed the animal more certainly than injury done to the posterior portion; but I found it difficult to make the experiment without injuring both portions.

Next, considering that the spinal nerves have a double root, and being of opinion that the properties of the nerves are derived from their connections with the parts of the brain, I thought that I had an opportunity of putting my opinion to the test of experiment, and of proving at the same time that nerves of different endowments were in the same cord, and held together by the same sheath.

On laying bare the roots of the spinal nerves, I found that I could cut across the posterior fasciculus of nerves, which took its origin from the posterior portion of the spinal marrow without convulsing the muscles of the back; but that on touching the anterior fasciculus with the point of a knife, the muscles of the back were immediately convulsed. Such were my reasons for concluding that the cerebrum and the cerebellum were parts distinct in function, and that every nerve possessing a double function obtained that by having a double root. I now saw the meaning of the double connection of the nerves with the spinal marrow; and also the cause of that seeming intricacy in the connections of nerves throughout their course, which were not double at their origins.

The spinal nerves being double, and having their roots in the spinal marrow, of which a portion comes from the cerebrum and a portion from the cerebellum, they convey the attributes of both grand divisions of the brain to every part; and therefore the distribution of such nerves is simple, one nerve supplying its distinct part. But the nerves which come directly from the brain, come from parts of the brain which vary in operation; and in order to bestow different qualities on the parts to which the nerves are distributed, two or more nerves must be united in their course or at their final destination. Hence it is that the first nerve must have branches of the fifth united with it: hence the *portio dura* of the seventh pervades every where the bones of the cranium to unite with the extended branches of the fifth: hence the union of the third and fifth in the orbit: hence the ninth and fifth are both sent to the tongue: hence it is, in short, that no part is sufficiently supplied by one single nerve, unless that nerve be a nerve of the spinal marrow, and have a double root, a connection (however remotely) with both the cerebrum and cerebellum. Such nerves as are single in their origin from the spinal marrow will be found either to unite in their course with some other nerve, or to be such as are acknowledged to be peculiar in their operation.

The eighth nerve is from the portion of the *medulla oblongata** which belongs to the cerebellum: the ninth nerve comes from the portion which belongs to

* The *medulla oblongata* is only the commencement of the spinal marrow.

the cerebrum. The first is a nerve of the class called Vital nerves, controlling secretly the operations of the body; the last is the motor nerve of the tongue, and is an instrument of volition. Now the connections formed by the eighth nerve in its course to the viscera are endless; it seems nowhere sufficient for the entire purpose of a nerve; for every where it is accompanied by others, and the ninth passes to the tongue, which is already profusely supplied by the fifth.

Understanding the origin of the nerves in the brain to be the source of their powers, we look upon the connections formed betwixt distant nerves, and upon the combination of nerves in their passage, with some interest; but without this, the whole is an unmeaning tissue. Seeing the seeming irregularity in one subject, we say it is accident; but finding that the connections never vary, we say only that it is strange, until we come to understand the necessity of nerves being combined in order to bestow distinct qualities on the parts to which they are sent.

The *cerebellum* when compared with the *cerebrum* is simple in its form. It has no internal tubercles or masses of cineritious matter in it. The medullary matter comes down from the cineritious cortex, and forms the *crus;* and the *crus* runs into union with the same process from the cerebrum; and they together form the *medulla spinalis,* and are continued down into the spinal marrow; and these crura or processes afford double origin to the double nerves of the spine.

THE NERVES PROCEEDING FROM THE CRUS CEREBELLI GO EVERY WHERE (IN SEEMING UNION WITH THOSE FROM THE CRUS CEREBRI) ; THEY UNITE THE BODY TOGETHER, AND CONTROUL THE ACTIONS OF THE BODILY FRAME ; AND ESPECIALLY GOVERN THE OPERATION OF THE VISCERA NECESSARY TO THE CONTINUANCE OF LIFE.

In all animals having a nervous system, the *cerebellum* is apparent, even though there be no *cerebrum.* The cerebrum is seen in such tribes of animals as have organs of sense, and it is seen to be near the eyes, or principal organ of sense; and sometimes it is quite separate from the *cerebellum.*

THE CEREBRUM I CONSIDER AS THE GRAND ORGAN BY WHICH THE MIND IS UNITED TO THE BODY. INTO IT ALL THE NERVES FROM THE EXTERNAL ORGANS OF THE SENSES ENTER; AND FROM IT ALL THE NERVES WHICH ARE AGENTS OF THE WILL PASS OUT.

If this be not at once obvious, it proceeds only from the circumstance that the nerves take their origin from the different parts of the brain ; and while those nerves are considered as simple cords, this circumstance stands opposed to the conclusion which otherwise would be drawn. A nerve having several roots implies that it propagates its sensation to the brain generally. But when we find that the several roots are distinct in their endowment, and are, in respect to office, distinct nerves; then the conclusion is unavoidable, that the portions of the brain are distinct organs of different functions.

To arrive at any understanding of the internal parts of the cerebrum, we must keep in view the relation of the nerves, and must class and distinguish the nerves, and follow them into its substance. If all ideas originate in the mind from external impulse, how can we better investigate the structure of the brain than by following the nerves, which are means of communication betwixt the brain and the outward organs of the senses?

The nerves of sense, the olfactory, the optic, the auditory, and the gustatory nerves, are traced backwards into certain tubercles or convex bodies in the base of the brain. And I may say, the nerves of sense either form tubercles before entering the brain, or they enter into those convexities in the base of the *cerebrum*. These convexities are the constituent parts of the cerebrum, and are in all animals necessary parts of the organs of sense; for as certainly as we discover an animal to have an external organ of sense, we find also a medullary tubercle; whilst the superiority of animals in intelligence is shown by the greater magnitude of the hemispheres or upper part of the cerebrum.

The convex bodies which are seated in the lower part of the cerebrum, and into which the nerves of sense enter, have extensive connection with the hemispheres on their upper part. FROM THE MEDULLARY

MATTER OF THE HEMISPHERES, *again, there pass down, converging to the crura, striæ, which is the medullary matter taking upon it the character of a nerve ; for from the crura cerebri, or its prolongation in the anterior fasciculi of the spinal marrow, go off* THE NERVES OF MOTION.

But WITH THESE NERVES OF MOTION *which are passing outward there are nerves going inwards ; nerves from the surfaces of the body ;* NERVES OF TOUCH ; AND NERVES OF PECULIAR SENSIBILITY, *having their seat in the body or viscera. It is not improbable that* THE TRACTS OF CINERITIOUS MATTER WHICH WE OBSERVE IN THE COURSE OF THE MEDULLARY MATTER OF THE BRAIN, ARE THE SEAT OF SUCH PECULIAR SENSIBILITIES ; *the organs of certain powers which seem resident in the body.*

As we proceed further in the investigation of the functions of the brain, the discussion becomes more hypothetical. But surely physiologists have been mistaken in supposing it necessary to prove sensibility in those parts of the brain which they are to suppose the seat of the intellectual operations. We are not to expect the same phenomena to result from the cutting or tearing of the brain as from the injury to the nerves. The function of the one is to transmit sensation ; the other has a higher operation. The nature of the organs of sense is different ; the sensibilities of the parts of the body are very various. If the needle piercing the retina during the operation of couching gives no remarkable pain, except in touching the common coats of the eye, ought we to imagine that the seat of the higher operations of the mind should, when injured, exhibit the same effects with the irritation of a nerve? So far therefore from thinking the parts of the brain which are insensible, to be parts inferior (as every part has its use), I should even from this be led to imagine that they had a higher office. And if there be certain parts of the brain which are insensible, and other parts which being injured shake the animal with convulsions exhibiting phenomena similar to those of a wounded nerve, it seems to follow that the latter parts which are endowed with sensibility like the nerves are similar to them in function and use; while the parts of the brain which possess no such sensibility are different in function and organization from the nerves, and have a distinct and higher operation to perform.

If in examining the apparent structure of the brain, we find a part consisting of white medullary striæ and fasciculated like a nerve, we should conclude that as the use of a nerve is to transmit sensation, not to perform any more peculiar function, such tracts of matter are media of communication, connecting the parts of the brain; rather than the brain itself performing the more peculiar functions. On the other hand, if masses are found in the brain unlike the matter of the nerve, and which yet occupy a place guarded as an organ of importance, we may presume that such parts have a use different from that of merely conveying sensation; we may rather look upon such parts as the seat of the higher powers.

Again, if those parts of the brain which are directly connected with the nerves, and which resemble them in structure, give pain when injured, and occasion convulsion to the animal as the nerves do when they are injured; and if, on the contrary, such parts as are more remote from the nerves, and of a different structure, produce no such effect when injured, we may conclude, that the office of the latter parts is more allied to the intellectual operations, less to mere sensation.

I have found at different times all the internal parts of the brain diseased without loss of sense; but I have never seen disease general on the surfaces of the hemispheres without derangement or oppression of the mind during the patient's life. In the case of derangement of mind, falling into lethargy or stupidity, I have constantly found the surface of the hemispheres dry and preternaturally firm, the membrane separating from it with unusual facility.

If I be correct in this view of the subject, then the experiments which have been made upon the brain tend to confirm the conclusions which I should be inclined to draw from strict anatomy; viz. that the cineritious and superficial parts of the brain are the seat of the intellectual functions. For it is found that the surface of the brain is totally insensible, but that the deep and medullary part being wounded, the animal is convulsed and pained.

At first it is difficult to comprehend how the part to which every sensation is referred, and by means of which we become acquainted with the various sensations, can itself be insensible; but the consideration of the wide difference of function betwixt a part destined to receive impressions, and a part which is the seat of intellect, reconciles us to the phenomenon. It would be rather strange to find that there were no distinction exhibited in experiments on parts evidently so different in function as the organs of the senses, the nerves, and the brain. Whether there be a difference in the matter of the nervous system, or a distinction in organization, is of so little importance to our enquiries, when it is proved that their essential properties are different, though their union and co-operation be necessary to the completion of their function—the development of the faculties by impulse from external matter.

All ideas originate in the brain: the operation producing them is the remote effect of an agitation or impression on the extremities of the nerves of sense; directly they are consequences of a change or operation in the proper organ of the SENSE *which constitutes a part of the* BRAIN, and over these organs, once brought into action by external impulse, the mind has influence. It is provided, that the extremities of the nerves of the senses shall be susceptible each of certain qualities in matter, and betwixt the impression of the outward sense, as it may be called, and the exercise of the internal organ, there is established a connection by which the ideas excited have a permanent correspondence with the qualities of bodies which surround us.

From the cineritious matter, which is chiefly external, and forming the surface of the cerebrum; and from the grand centre of medullary matter of the cerebrum, what are called the crura descend. These are fasciculated processes of the CEREBRUM, *from which go off the nerves of* MOTION, the nerves governing the muscular frame. Through the nerves of sense, the *sensorium* receives impressions, but the will is expressed through the medium of the nerves of motion. THE SECRET OPERATIONS OF THE BODILY FRAME, AND THE CONNECTIONS WHICH UNITE THE PARTS OF THE BODY INTO A SYSTEM, ARE THROUGH THE CEREBELLUM AND NERVES PROCEEDING FROM IT.

EXTRACTS FROM

SKETCH OF A GENERAL THEORY OF THE INTELLECTUAL FACULTIES OF MAN AND ANIMALS,

GIVEN IN REPLY TO DRS. CROSS AND LEACH.

BY ALEXANDER WALKER.

Date of Publication—July, 1815.

From Dr. Thomson's Annals of Philosophy for July, 1815, *Article VI.*

* * * * * *

I NOW state some of my reasons for asserting, that the organs of sense being those of sensation, and the cerebrum that of mental operation, the cerebellum is the organ of volition, or rather of all the motions of animals, voluntary and involuntary.

1. There are *three distinct intellectual organs* or classes of intellectual organs, namely, the organs of sense, the cerebrum, and the cerebellum That the cerebellum, though separated from the cerebrum only by membranes in man, is not on that account less distinct from it than are the organs of sense separated by bony plates, is rendered evident by the consideration, that membranes form in one case, as effectual a separation as bony plates do in the other; that many

animals* have a bony tentorium between the cerebrum and cerebellum, as they have bony plates between the cerebrum and face; and that others (birds) have membranes between the cerebrum and face, as they have a membranous tentorium between the cerebrum and cerebellum.

2. There are *three distinct intellectual functions* or classes of intellectual functions, namely, sensation, mental operation,† and volition.

3. Of the *organs*, those of the senses are the first, the cerebrum intermediate, and the *cerebellum the last.* For, although the face, containing the organs of sense, and the cerebellum, are, in different animals, very differently placed with regard to the cerebrum, yet there is a peculiar relation between the situation of one of these and that of the others with regard to it. In other words, although the face is sometimes in one situation and sometimes in another with relation to the cerebrum, yet to each given variation of its situation with regard to that body there is a corresponding and uniformly accompanying variation in the situation of the cerebellum. Thus as, in man, the face is placed below the anterior part of the cerebrum, so is the cerebellum placed below its posterior part; and precisely as, in the inferior animals, the face advances, precisely so does the cerebellum re-

* Viz. most species of the cat and bear kind, the martin *(mustela martes)*, the coaita *(ceropithecus paniscus)*, and others.

† Including observation, reflection, judgment, and subordinate faculties.

cede, till, in those animals in which the face is placed exactly before the cerebrum, the cerebellum is placed exactly behind it.*

4. Of the *functions*, sensation is the first, mental operation intermediate, and *volition the last.* That sensation precedes and excites, if it do not generate, mental operation, few will deny: that mental operation, however rapid or evanescent, precedes and excites volition, or that the motive to an action must precede the action, none will refuse: and that, of any one series of intellectual action, volition is the last stage, all must admit.

5. As, then, the *cerebellum* is the last of the intellectual *organs*, and *volition* the last of the intellectual *functions*, and as, at the same time, there is no organ without function, or function without organ, it follows, that the cerebellum must be the organ of volition.

6. In perfect conformity with this truth, the inferior animals, however defective in intellect, possess motion; and in almost all of them which have any visible nervous system, a cerebellum, the organ of that motion, exists.—This leads me to an observation which seems to me to possess considerable interest and beauty. As we descend among animals, one of the three portions of the nervous system and one of its three general functions gradually disappear. Now it is not the first and the last portions of the nervous

* The cerebellic cavity, moreover, seems uniformly to commence on the inside of the base of the cranium exactly opposite to the place where the face, or the lower jaw, terminates on the outside.

system — it is not the organs of sense and the cerebellum, neither is it their respective functions, sensation and volition, which are thus lost. It is the cerebrum and mental operation which are. This organ is, among men, most conspicuous in the Caucasian race; and we accordingly find that that race alone has cultivated the sciences. It is less even in the Mongol and Ethiop, who have ever disregarded them. It gradually disappears and ultimately evanishes as we descend among quadrupeds, birds, reptiles, fishes, &c. and with it gradually disappear and ultimately evanish the powers of thought. But organs of sense and a cerebellum,—sensation and volition, yet remain to characterize myriads of animals below these.

7. This truth receives new confirmation when we observe, that the degrees of voluntary power always bear a close analogy to the various magnitudes of the cerebellum. In fishes, for instance, which possess amazing locomotive power, the cerebellum is often larger than the cerebrum; and they sometimes possess an additional tubercle, which seems to Cuvier to form a second cerebellum! *

* * * * * *

* NOTE REDUCED FROM TEXT. — Dr. Cross says "that volition ranks among the faculties of the mind, whose organ is the cerebrum;" and "that affections of the cerebrum, while the cerebellum remains sound, produce palsy, which I humbly submit is just a loss of volition." Hence he means to conclude that palsy, which he deems a loss of volition, and consequently volition itself, are dependent on the cerebrum, and not on the cerebellum: indeed, he actually says so in the preceding portion of the same

CONCLUSION OF THE SAME PAPER.

[*From the same Journal for August*, 1815, *Article VI.*]

On the subject of the cerebellum, I have only to add, that all the observations which Drs. Gall and Spurzheim have adduced to prove that it is the organ of amativeness, are accountable from the circumstance that the degree of physical love seems to be more or less connected with the degree of voluntary power—the proper function of this organ: and hence it is that the man, the stallion, and the bull, having more voluntary power, have also more amativeness, and a larger cerebellum than the eunuch, the gelding, and the ox.

My former brief paper being entitled, On the Use of the Cerebellum and Spinal Marrow, it was less to the structure of these parts (which I conceive to be sufficiently well-known) than to their use that I

sentence. The conclusion, however, is inaccurate ; for even, if palsy were just a loss of volition, it would be by no means wonderful if the functions of the cerebellum were deranged by an injury of the cerebrum, since two immediately contiguous and intimately connected organs must powerfully influence each other. Dr. Cross must be aware that even remote organs evidence this sympathy. Thus, no derangement of volition, caused by injury of the cerebrum, is any proof that the cerebrum is the seat of volition. He humbly submits that palsy is just a loss of volition. I reply that palsy is no such thing ; and as the Dr. is fond of logic, I shall give him my proof in logical form.—We cannot be conscious of any mental act unless that act exist: but volition is a mental act of which the patient is conscious in palsy: therefore palsy is not just a loss of volition!

referred. In particular * * * it was my intention to consider as my own, the observation that the anterior columns (in which end the anterior spinal nerves) terminate in the cerebrum, while the posterior columns (in which begin the posterior spinal nerves) commence in the cerebellum; as well as that the anterior may be termed the ascending columns and nerves, and the posterior the descending—that the former may be called those of sensation or impression, which, to be cognizable to the brain, must ascend from by far the greater part of the surface of the body; and that the posterior may be called those of volition or expression, which, to affect almost all the muscles, must descend from the head. And, to say the least of it, this is rendered highly probable by the circumstances that sensation and volition—an ascending and a descending motion cannot possibly take place in the same fibrils of the same nerve; that consequently all nerves, having at once sensation and volition, divide into two series of fibrils on joining the spinal marrow, namely, an anterior series and a posterior one; that the anterior series is, in form and structure, totally different from the posterior; and that the spinal marrow, divided as it is by fissures and by cineritious matter, does really form four columns which are joined by these series, viz. the anterior columns, by the anterior fasciculi, and the posterior columns, by the posterior fasciculi.

* * * * * *

In replying to my statement, that the anterior of the nervous fasciculi which join the spinal marrow, are not nerves of sensation, nor the posterior nerves of volition, Dr. Leach, instead of proving my inaccuracy, places upon record a most astonishing specimen of his own! Dr. Leach says, "The two roots of nerves of each half of the spinal marrow, namely, the anterior and posterior, go to different parts of the body:—the muscles and skin of the back receive their nerves from the posterior roots, whilst the muscles and skin of the abdomen receive theirs from the anterior roots, and yet the fore and back parts of the body have sensation and voluntary motion." Now certainly if this were but true, my doctrine would be not merely inaccurate, but altogether false; for this would prove, that both roots were at once nerves of sensation and of volition: but, not being true, the case is certainly somewhat altered. Unluckily for Dr. Leach, it is his own statement which is inaccurate. In his "careful examination of the structure of the spinal mass of nerves," the Dr. has absolutely mistaken the *branches* for the *roots* of these nerves! It is from the branches that the nerves he alludes to go off; for, however lucky this may be for humanity, since it prevents our moving with only one half the body, and feeling only with the other, it is certainly unfortunate for the Dr.'s argument, that neither to skin nor muscles is the slightest twig given from the roots. These roots then combine, communicate, and even cross by twigs, in order to form a trunk; and, that the Dr. may not be put to the trouble of another "careful examination," *if he will only cross the fingers of one of his hands between those of the other, he will have a tolerable conception of the trunk so formed, remembering, however, that only about half the fibrils of either root do so cross, while the other half, instead of crossing to the opposite branch, runs onward in the branch of the same side.* A rather greater number of fibrils, indeed, pass from the posterior root to the anterior branch than from the anterior root to the posterior branch, because the anterior branch, being destined to supply a greater portion of the body, requires to be larger. *I do not find this decussation described in any anatomical book,* which I have at hand; but the slightest inspection will demonstrate it. The law of this decussation is maintained even in very inferior animals; for, in those which have no vertebræ and in which the spinal marrow is formed below the œsophagus by the union of the two crura of the cerebellum, though the two fasciculi generally remain distinct throughout the greater part of their length, yet they always unite at different spaces by knots whenever a nerve is given off! Thus *each branch* is composed from *both roots:* and it is only from the branches thus *composed,* and by no mean from the roots, that the nerves the Dr. speaks of are distributed: hence it is not wonderful that they give both sensation and voluntary motion. These *branches,* however, the Doctor calls "the two *roots of nerves of each half of the spinal marrow*, namely, the anterior and posterior;" and asserts, as is seen above, that these identical ROOTS of *each half* of the spinal marrow "go to different parts of the body!" Every anatomist and every anatomical work declares that from the roots no twig proceeds either to skin or muscles; and if it were not obvious that the Doctor had mistaken the branches for the roots, I should be apt to think that, in his "careful examination of the structure of the spinal mass of nerves," the Doctor had refuted the whole of them.

* * * * * *

In proof, however, that the sensitive and motive nerves are perfectly distinct, I can quote for Dr. Leach a much better authority than that of any old author: *first, that of reason, which tells us, that as sensation cannot reach the cerebrum without an ascending motion—a motion towards the brain; as the consequent volition cannot affect the muscles without a descending motion—a motion from the brain; and as it is contrary to all analogy that there should be motion in opposite directions in the same tubes of neurilema—for these reasons, there must be a series of nerves appropriated to each: and secondly, the authority of anatomy, which shews us that, though nerves supplying parts which are contiguous in position but different in nature often run in one common sheath, yet, on arriving at the spinal marrow, they split into two roots, as they are termed; that these roots are quite different in form, the anterior being more fibrous, and the posterior more simple and round; that the anterior roots join the anterior columns of the spinal marrow, and the posterior roots the posterior columns; that these columns actually do join the cerebrum and cerebellum respectively; and that even those cerebral nerves which are at once nerves of sensation and volition have two roots, one from the cerebrum, and another from the cerebellum.* This may be most easily observed in the seventh pair or facial nerves.

* * * * * *

The leading heads, then, of this new system of the intellectual functions are as follows:—

1. THAT THE NERVES OF SENSATION ARISE IN THE ORGANS OF SENSE, AND, BY MEANS OF THE ANTERIOR FIBRILS, TERMINATE IN THE ANTERIOR COLUMNS OF THE SPINAL MARROW.

2. THAT THOSE NERVES OF SENSATION WHICH DO NOT TERMINATE IN THESE COLUMNS, PASS DIRECTLY TO THE CEREBRUM.

3. THAT THE ANTERIOR COLUMNS OF THE SPINAL MARROW TERMINATE ALSO IN THE ANTERIOR PART OF THE CEREBRUM.

4. THAT THESE NERVES AND COLUMNS ARE THE SENSITIVE OR ASCENDING NERVES AND COLUMNS.

5. THAT IT IS IN THIS WAY THAT SENSATION BECOMES PERCEPTION, AND THAT ARE EXCITED IN THE CEREBRUM THE FACULTIES, &c.

6. THAT THE CEREBRAL INFLUENCE PASSES TO THE CEREBELLUM BY MEANS OF THE CORPORA STRIATA POSTERIORA OR THALAMI, THE ANTERIOR PEDUNCLES OF THE CEREBELLUM, &c.

7. THAT THE CEREBELLUM IS THE ORGAN WHICH GIVES IMPULSE TO ALL MUSCULAR MOTION, VOLUNTARY AND INVOLUNTARY (subsequently corrected as to the latter).

8. THAT THE POSTERIOR COLUMNS OF THE SPINAL MARROW ORIGINATE IN THE CEREBELLUM.

9. THAT FROM THE CEREBELLUM ARISE ALSO SEVERAL NERVES OF VOLITION.

10. THAT THOSE NERVES OF VOLITION WHICH DO NOT ARISE DIRECTLY FROM THE CEREBELLUM, SPRING FROM THE POSTERIOR COLUMNS OF THE SPINAL MARROW BY MEANS OF THE POSTERIOR FIBRILS.

11. THAT THESE NERVES AND COLUMNS ARE THE MOTIVE OR DESCENDING NERVES AND COLUMNS.

12. * * * THAT THE INTENSITY OF THE INTELLECTUAL FUNCTIONS IS AS THE LENGTH OF THEIR ORGANS, AND THE PERMANENCE OF THESE FUNCTIONS AS THE BREADTH OF THEIR ORGANS.

I believe that none of these statements were ever made by any one before they were made either here or elsewhere by myself; but should *any* of them have been previously made on any rational ground, I shall feel no pain in resigning the merit or demerit of their discovery to its proper author. Still less, of course, has the general system which I now advance been thought of by any one.

It appears, then, that THERE IS A SPECIES OF CIRCULATION IN THE NERVOUS SYSTEM, OF WHICH I HAVE SKETCHED THE GENERAL COURSE, AS CURIOUS AND ADMIRABLE AS THAT WHICH EXISTS IN THE

VASCULAR (THE CENTRE OF THE ONE BEING THE HEART, AND OF THE OTHER THE HEAD); AND THAT THERE IS SCARCELY ANY POINT OF THE BODY WHICH THIS CIRCLE DOES NOT INVOLVE AND REST ON, SINCE FROM ALMOST EVERY POINT ASCENDS IMPRESSION TO THE CEREBRUM BY A NERVE OF SENSATION, THE ANTERIOR NERVOUS ROOTS, AND THE ANTERIOR COLUMNS OF THE SPINAL MARROW; AND TO EACH RETURNS EXPRESSION FROM THE CEREBELLUM BY THE POSTERIOR COLUMNS, THE POSTERIOR NERVOUS ROOTS, AND THE NERVES OF VOLITION.

EXTRACTS FROM A PAPER

ON THE NERVES; GIVING AN ACCOUNT OF SOME EXPERIMENTS ON THEIR STRUCTURE AND FUNCTIONS,

WHICH LEAD TO A NEW ARRANGEMENT OF THE SYSTEM.

BY CHARLES BELL, Esq.

Date. — *Read to the Royal Society, July* 12, 1821.

This paper is extracted from Philosophical Transactions of the Royal Society of London, for the year 1821, *Part* II. *Vol.* 110 & 111.

* * * * * *

OBJECT OF THE PAPER.—The Author means to limit his present enquiry to *the nerves of respiration.*

[*Having given this statement from the paper itself, the Editor need scarcely add that it contains not one word relating to sensation and volition as respectively the functions of anterior or posterior spinal nerves, spinal columns, and cerebral masses. It is inserted in consequence of what is said in it of the trifacial and facial nerves, and of the mere analogy supposed to exist between these and the spinal nerves, notwithstanding the acknow-*

ledged fact that the posterior spinal nerves are either *sensitive or motory, while the ganglionic portion of the trifacial is* both *sensitive, and, as Bellingeri has shown, involuntarily motory. The existence of a ganglion certainly can prove nothing till the use of a ganglion is known.*]

THE NERVES ARE DIVIDED INTO TWO PARTS OR SYSTEMS; ONE SIMPLE AND UNIFORM, &c. * * * Where an animal is endowed with mere sensation and locomotion, where there is no central organ of circulation, and no organ of respiration but what is generally diffused over the frame, the nerves are extremely simple; they consist of two cords running in the length of the body, with branches going off laterally to the several divisions of the frame. And here no intricacy is to be seen, no double supply of nerves is to be observed, but each portion of the frame has an equal supply; and the central line of connection is sufficient to combine the actions of the muscles, and to give them the concatenation necessary to locomotion.

There is the same uniform and symmetrical system of nerves in the human body as in the leech or worm; although obscured by a variety of superadded nerves. These additional nerves belong to organs, which, tracing the orders of animals upward, are observed gradually to accumulate until we arrive at the complication of the human frame. These nerves, additional and superadded to the original system, do not destroy, but only obscure that system; and accordingly, when we separate certain nerves, the original system of simple constitution is presented even in the human body.

The nerves of the spine, the tenth or sub-occipital nerve, and the fifth or trigeminus of the system of Willis, constitute this original and symmetrical system. All these nerves agree in these essential circumstances; they have all double origins; they have all ganglia on one of their roots; they go out laterally to certain divisions of the body; they do not interfere to unite the divisions of the frame; *they are all muscular nerves, ordering the voluntary motions of the frame; they are all exquisitely sensible, and the source of the common sensibility of the surfaces of the body;* when accurately represented on paper, they are seen to pervade every part; no part is without them; and yet they are symmetrical and simple as the nerves of the lower animals.

If the nerves be exposed in a living animal, those of this class exhibit the highest degree of sensibility; while, on the contrary, nerves not of this original class or system, are comparatively so little sensible, as to be immediately distinguished; in so much that the quiescence of the animal suggests a doubt whether they be sensible in any degree whatever. If the *fifth nerve,* and *the portio dura of the seventh,* be both exposed on the face of a living animal, there will not remain the slightest doubt in the mind of the experimenter which of these nerves bestows sensibility. If the nerve of this original class be divided, the skin and common substance is deprived of sensibility; but if a nerve not of this class be divided, it in no measure deprives the parts of their sensibility to external impression.

MORE PARTICULARLY OF THE RESPIRATORY NERVES. —The nerves which connect the internal organs of respiration with the sensibilities of remote parts, and with the respiratory muscles, are distinguished from those of which we have been speaking by many circumstances. They do not arise by double roots; they have no ganglia on their origins; they come off from the *medulla oblongata* and the upper part of the spinal marrow; and from this origin, they diverge to those several remote parts of the frame which are combined in the motion of respiration. These are the nerves which give the appearance of confusion to the dissection, because they cross the others, and go to parts already plentifully supplied from the other system.

The following are the nerves to be enumerated, as *respiratory nerves,* according to their functions: [enumeration abridged] — 1. *Par vagum,* the eighth of Willis, the *pneumo-gastric nerve* of the modern French physiologists; 2. *Respiratory nerve of the face,* being that which is called *portio dura* of the seventh; 3. *Superior respiratory nerve of the trunk,* being that which is called *spinal accessory;* 4. *Great internal respiratory nerve*—the *phrenic* or *diaphragmatic,* of authors; 5. *The external respiratory nerve:* this has a similar origin with the preceding nerve.

These four last-mentioned nerves govern the muscles of the face, neck, shoulders, and chest, in the actions of excited respiration, and are absolutely necessary to speech and expression. But there are other nerves of the same class which go to the tongue, throat, and windpipe, no less essential to complete the act of respiration. These are the glosso-pharyngeal nerve, the lingual, or ninth of Willis, and the branches of the par vagum to the superior and inferior larynx.

Of the nerves of the face, in which it is shown that the two sets of nerves, hitherto supposed to be similar, differ in structure, sensibility, and function.— * * * The nerves of the face are, first, the *trigeminus*, or the 5th of Willis, and that familiarly called the *portio dura* of the seventh, but which, in this paper, will be called *the respiratory nerve of the face.*

The trigeminus, or fifth pair.— * * * *It is the nerve of taste and of the salivary glands; of the muscles of the face and jaws, and of common sensibility.* This nerve comes off from the base of the brain in so peculiar a situation, that it alone, of all the nerves of the head, receives *roots both from the medullary process of the cerebrum and of the cerebellum.* A ganglion is formed upon it near its origin, though some of its filaments pass on without entering into the ganglion. Before passing out of the skull the nerve splits into three great divisions, which are sent to the face, jaws and tongue. *Its branches go* *minutely into the skin and enter into* ALL *the muscles, and they are especially profuse to the muscles which move the lips upon the teeth.**

THE RESPIRATORY NERVE OF THE FACE, being that which is called portio dura of the seventh.—This nerve does not exist except where there is some consent of motions established betwixt the face and the respiratory organs. * * *

The respiratory nerve of the face arises from the superior and lateral part of the *medulla oblongata*, close to the *nodus cerebri*, and exactly where the *crus cerebelli* joins the *medulla oblongata*. The other respiratory nerves, which form so distinguished a part of the nervous system, arise in a line with the roots of this. * * *

While within the temporal bone, two cords of communication are formed with the branches of the fifth nerve, or *trigeminus*. One of these is called Vidian nerve, and the other *corda tympani*. By these communications, nerves go in both directions; branches of the seventh are sent to the membrane of the nose, and to the muscles at the back of the palate; while branches of the fifth nerve (and also of

* In a note in the third edition, the author here adds—"I have often been requested, in vindication of the correctness of my *original* account of the fifth nerve, to report my early statement of the uses of this nerve. I can give nothing more distinct than in this passage."—This, now before the reader, is a literal transcript of the *original* account. Its uses, as originally indicated, are further detailed under the head of "Experiments," &c. and of "Function of the Trigeminus."

the sympathetic nerve) are brought into the interior of the ear.

By the second of these communications, the *corda tympani* (which joins the lingual branch of the fifth, just where that nerve is passing by the side of the *levator* and *circumflexus palati*), the branches of this respiratory nerve have access to the *velum palati* and its muscles.

The respiratory nerve of the face, emerging through the stylomastoid foramen, divides into many branches, and these diverging, spread to all the side of the face. First, a branch is sent to the muscles of the outward ear; another is sent, under the angle of the jaw, to the muscles of the throat. The principal nerve then passes through the parotid gland and comes upon the face. Here the branches continue to scatter, to go upwards upon the temple, and downwards upon the side of the neck, forming on the neck a superficial plexus. The principal branches, however, go forward to the muscles of the forehead and eyelids; a branch called superior facial is sent to the muscles of the cheek and the side of the nose; while an inferior facial branch is given to the angle of the mouth and the muscles which concentrate there.

In this extensive distribution, *the nerve penetrates to* ALL *the muscles of the face; muscles, supplied also with the branches of the fifth pair. Its branches penetrate to the skin, accompanying the minute vessels of the cheek.*

The descending or inferior divisions, which go

under the lower jaw and to the superficial muscles of the throat and neck, are connected with branches of the spinal nerves, and with the respiratory nerves.

When we minutely observe the texture of the respiratory nerve of the face, we find it to correspond with the structure of the par vagum and to differ from that of the trigeminus. The filaments of this nerve have a very close texture, like a minute plexus. The fifth, compared to it, has large free round filaments with less intricacy in their texture.

If we were barely to consider this distribution of the *portio dura* of the seventh, unbiassed by theory or opinion, we should be forced to conclude, that it is not alone sufficient to supply any one part with nervous power, for every one of its branches is joined by divisions of the fifth. The question then naturally arises, whether these nerves perform the same function? whether they furnish a double supply of the same property or endowment, or whether they do not perform different offices? * * *

Experiments on the nerves of the face.—An ass being thrown, and its nostrils confined for a few seconds, so as to make it pant and forcibly dilate the nostrils at each inspiration, the *portio dura was divided on one side of the head;* the motion of the nostril of the same side instantly ceased, while the other nostril continued to expand and contract in unison with the motions of the chest.

On the division of the nerve, the animal gave no

sign of pain; there was no struggle nor effort made when it was cut across.

The animal being untied and corn and hay given to him, *he ate without the slightest impediment.*

An ass being tied and thrown, the superior maxillary branch of the fifth nerve was exposed. Touching this nerve gave acute pain. It was divided: but no change took place in the motion of the nostril; the cartilages continued to expand regularly in time with the other parts which combine in the act of respiration; but *the side of the lip was observed to hang low, and it was dragged to the other side.* The same branch of the fifth was divided on the opposite side, and the animal let loose. He could no longer pick up his corn; *the power of elevating and projecting the lip, as in gathering food, was lost.* To open the lips the animal pressed the mouth against the ground, and at length licked the oats from the ground with his tongue. *The loss of motion of the lips in eating was so obvious,* that it was thought a useless cruelty to cut the other branches of the fifth.

This experiment of cutting the respiratory nerve of the face, or *portio dura,* gave so little pain, that it was several times repeated on the ass and dog, and uniformly with the same effect. The side of the face remained at rest and placid, during the highest excitement of the other parts of the respiratory organs. * * *

When an animal becomes insensible from loss of blood, the impression at the heart extends its influence in violent convulsions over all the muscles of respiration; not only is the air drawn into the chest with sudden and powerful effort, but at the same instant the muscles of the mouth, nostrils and eye-lids, and all the side of the face, are in a violent state of spasm. In the ass, where the respiratory nerve of the face had been cut, the most remarkable contrast was exhibited in the two sides of its face; for whilst the one side was in universal and powerful contraction, the other, where the nerve was divided, remained quite placid.

From these facts we are entitled to conclude, that the *portio dura* of the seventh, is the respiratory nerve of the face; and that *the motions of the lips, the nostrils, and the velum palati are governed by its influence, when the muscles of these parts are in associated action with the other organs of respiration.* * * *

The actions of sneezing and coughing are entirely confined to the influence of the respiratory nerves. When carbonate of ammonia was put to the nostrils of the ass whose respiratory nerve had been cut, that side of the nose and face where the nerves were entire, was curled up with the peculiar expression of sneezing; but on the other side, where the nerve was divided, the face remained quite relaxed, although the branches of the fifth pair and the sympathetic were entire. The respiratory nerve of one side of the face of the dog being cut, the same effect was produced; the action of sneezing was entirely confined to one side of the face.

These last experiments show, that the peculiar expression in sneezing, results from *an impression on the respiratory nerves*, and that the muscles of the face are drawn into sympathy solely by the influence of the respiratory nerve of the face.*

* * * * *

We have proofs equal to experiments, that in the human face the actions of the muscles which produce smiling and laughing, are a consequence of the influence of this respiratory nerve. * * *

Thus it appears, that whenever the action of any of the muscles of the face is associated with the act of breathing, it is performed through the operation of this nerve. * * *

Function of the trigeminus, or fifth nerve, as illustrated by these experiments.—*We have seen that when the fifth nerve, the nerve of mastication and sensation, was cut in an ass, the animal could no longer gather his food. In the individual whose face was paralyzed on one side during the excited state of the respiratory organs, there could be observed no debility or paralysis in the same muscles when he took a morsel into his mouth, and began to chew.*

By an experiment made on the 16th of March, it was found, that on cutting the infra-orbitary branch of the fifth nerve on the left side, and the *portio dura*,

* Still making this a nerve of impression, Sir C. Bell, in his third edition adds, "It will appear that the property of receiving impression is not actually lost by the division of this facial muscular nerve, but the corresponding expression is quite destroyed."

or respiratory, on the right side of an ass, the sensibility to pain on the right side, where the *portio dura* of the seventh nerve was cut, remained entire, while that of the left side was completely destroyed by the division of the fifth. * * * The cutting of the fifth nerve gave pain in a degree corresponding with our notions of the sensibility of nerves; but in cutting the *portio dura*, it was not evident that the animal suffered pain at all.

Independently of the difference of sensibility in these nerves, there was exhibited, in all these experiments a wide distinction in their powers of exciting the muscles. The slightest touch on the *portio dura*, or respiratory nerve, convulsed the muscles of the face, whilst the animal gave no signs of pain. *By means of the branches of the fifth nerve, it was more difficult to produce any degree of action in the muscles*, although, as I have said, touching the nerve gave great pain.

I divided the branch of the fifth pair, which goes to the forehead, in a man, at his urgent request, on account of the *tic doloureux:* there followed no paralysis of the muscles of the eyebrow; but in an individual where an ulcer and abscess seated anterior to the tube of the ear affected the superior branch of the respiratory nerve, the eyebrow fell low, and did not follow the other when the features were animated by discourse or emotion.

* * * * *

NOTE ON THIS PAPER BY THE EDITOR.

The Editor has hitherto carefully avoided remarks on the subjects of these papers. He must notice, however, that the extracts from this paper are made from it as it originally appeared in the Philosophical Transactions. But as new editions of it have been published, and as in these editions, while retaining the original date of 1821, new matters have been introduced, *he must either submit to the injury of having the present copy of it stigmatized as incorrect, or he must vindicate himself by showing that* the subsequent editions, while retaining the original date, have really had new views introduced.—*As the whole object of this work is to supply original documents, he is compelled to choose the latter alternative.*

These surreptitious additions, that is, additions of new matter while the old date is retained, do, it must be acknowledged, by giving a false appearance of anticipation, unjustly tend to deprive Messrs. Magendie and Mayo of their unquestionable priority on some most important points.

In page 48 *of the third edition, speaking of the nerve of the* 5*th pair, Sir C. Bell says, "It alone, of all the nerves of the head, receives roots both from* the column of sensibility and from that of motion"—*substituting these last words for the original expression* "the medullary process of the cerebrum and of the cerebellum." *Now, the medullary processes of the cerebrum and of the cerebellum are not the columns of the spinal marrow; nor, in the original expression, is either sensibility or motion imputed to these medullary processes!* This altered expression, then, appears to anticipate Magendie's distinction in 1822 of these columns, as well as of the spinal roots, into posterior sensory and anterior motory. *But as this is in reality* a mere interpolation appearing much later than Magendie's paper did, *it tends to do him great injustice.* A PAPER SO ALTERED AS THIS IS, CANNOT HONOURABLY BE REPUBLISHED WITH THE DATE OF 1821.

In a note introduced in the third edition from a paper by Mr. John Shaw, a comparison is made between the 5th pair and the spinal nerves. But from this no conclusion as to priority can be drawn in favour of Sir C. Bell, because there is no proof of its having appeared in any form at this early period.—Other notes have a similar tendency to seem to anticipate.

In the text of this paper, as well as in various other notes in the third edition, Sir C. Bell's opinions as to the 5th and 7th pairs of nerves are greatly modified. But this affords no conclusion as to priority, because, as indeed all the world now knows, these modifications were the direct and immediate though unacknowledged results of Mr. Mayo's previous corrections.

The only other paper of Sir C. Bell, preceding Magendie's celebrated "Expériences," published in August, 1822, *and October of the same year, is Sir C. Bell's—" Of the nerves which associate the muscles of the chest, in the actions of breathing, speaking and expression ; being a continuation of the paper on the structure and functions of the nerves ;" read to the Royal Society, May* 2, 1822.

*There, he observes, that " In a former paper an examination was made of the nerves of the face ; that part of the system was taken, as proving in a manner the least liable to exception, that two sets of nerves, hitherto undistinguished, possessed distinct powers ; and that very different effects were produced when the muscles and integuments were deprived of the controlling influence of the one or of the other of these nerves. * * * In the present paper, it is proposed to prosecute this subject, by tracing the nerves which influence the motions of the trunk of the body in respiration, and to subject them to a similar enquiry."*

The paper contains not one word relating to sensation and volition as respectively the functions of anterior or posterior spinal nerves, spinal columns, and cerebral masses ; and it therefore left the field open for

EXPÉRIENCES SUR LES FONCTIONS DES RACINES DES NERFS RACHIDIENS.

PAR F. MAGENDIE,

MEMBRE DE L'INSTITUT DE FRANCE, ETC.

Date of Publication—1822.

Journal de Physiologie Expérimentale et Pathologique.
3e *Numéro.* *Août*, 1822.

DEPUIS long-temps je désirais faire une expérience dans laquelle je couperais sur un animal, les racines postérieures des nerfs qui naissent de la moëlle épinière. Je l'avais tentée bien des fois, sans pouvoir y réussir, à cause de la difficulté d'ouvrir le canal vertébral sans léser la moëlle, et par suite sans faire périr ou tout au moins sans blesser grièvement l'animal.

EXPERIMENTS UPON THE FUNCTIONS OF THE ROOTS OF THE SPINAL NERVES,

BY F. MAGENDIE, MEMBER OF THE INSTITUTE OF FRANCE, ETC.

Journal of Physiology Experimental and Pathological, No. III., *August*, 1822.

I HAD long been desirous of making the experiment of dividing in an animal the posterior roots of the nerves which arise from the spinal marrow. I had several times made the attempt, without being able to succeed, on account of the difficulty of opening the vertebral canal without injuring the spinal marrow, and consequently without destroying or at least seriously wounding the animal. Last month

Le mois dernier, on apporta dans mon laboratoire, une portée de huit petits chiens, âgés de six semaines; ces animaux me parurent très-propres à tenter de nouveau d'ouvrir le canal vertébral. En effet, je pus à l'aide d'un scalpel bien tranchant, et pour ainsi dire d'un seul coup, mettre à nu la moitié postérieure de la moëlle épinière entourée de ses enveloppes. Il ne me restait pour avoir cet organe presqu'à nu, que de couper la dure-mère qui l'entoure : c'est ce que je fis avec facilité ; j'eus alors sous les yeux les racines postérieures des paires lombaires et sacrées, et en les soulevant successivement avec les lames de petits ciseaux, je pus les couper d'un côté, la moëlle restant intacte. J'ignorais quel serait le résultat de cette tentative; je réunis la plaie par une suture à la peau, et j'observai l'animal; je crus d'abord le membre correspondant aux nerfs coupés, entièrement paralysé ; il était insensible aux piqûres et aux pressions les plus

---

there was brought to my laboratory a litter of eight puppies, six weeks old; these animals appeared to me very suitable for a new attempt at opening the vertebral canal. I was able indeed, with the help of a very sharp scalpel, and I may say at a single cut, to expose the posterior half of the spinal marrow surrounded by its envelopes. There only remained for the complete exposure of this organ to cut the dura-mater which surrounds it: this I did with facility; I then had a complete view of the posterior roots of the lumbar and sacral pairs, and in lifting them up successively with the points of a small pair of scissors, I was able to cut them on one side, the spinal marrow remaining untouched. I was ignorant what might be the result of this attempt; I reunited the wound by a suture, and then observed the animal; I at first thought the member corresponding to the cut nerves, was entirely paralysed; it was insensible to the strongest prickings and pressures, it seemed to me also incapable

fortes, il me paraissait aussi immobile ; mais bientôt, à ma grande surprise, je le vis se mouvoir d'une manière très-apparente, bien que la sensibilité y fût toujours tout-à-fait éteinte. Une seconde, une troisième expérience, me donnèrent exactement le même résultat ; je commençai à regarder comme probable que les racines postérieures des nerfs rachidiens pourraient bien avoir des fonctions différentes des racines antérieures, et qu'elles étaient plus particulièrement destinées à la sensibilité.

Il se présentait naturellement à l'esprit de couper les racines antérieures, en laissant intactes les postérieures ; mais une semblable entreprise était plus facile à concevoir qu'à exécuter ; comment mettre à découvert la partie antérieure de la moëlle, sans intéresser les racines postérieures ? J'avoue que la chose me parut d'abord impossible ; cependant je ne cessai d'y rêver pendant deux jours, et enfin je me décidai à essayer de passer devant les racines postérieures,

---

of moving; but soon, to my great surprise, I saw it move in a manner very apparent, although sensibility was entirely extinct. A second and third experiment gave me exactly the same result; I began to think it probable that the posterior roots of the spinal nerves might have different functions from the anterior roots, and that they were more particularly destined for sensation.

It naturally occurred to the mind to cut the anterior roots, leaving the posterior untouched; but such an enterprise was more easily conceived than executed; how expose the anterior part of the spinal marrow, without interfering with the posterior roots? I confess that the thing at first appeared to me to be impossible; nevertheless for two days I continued to think of it, and at last I decided to endeavour to pass before the posterior roots, a sort of cataract knife,

une espèce de couteau à cataracte, dont la lame, très-étroite, permettrait de pouvoir couper les racines, en les pressant avec le tranchant de l'instrument, sur la face postérieure du corps des vertèbres; mais je fus obligé de renoncer à cette manœuvre, à cause des grosses veines que contient le canal de ce côté, et que j'ouvrais à chaque mouvement en avant. En faisant ces essais, je m'aperçus qu'en tirant sur la dure-mère vertébrale, on pouvait entrevoir les racines antérieures réunies en faisceaux, au moment où elles vont percer cette membrane. Il ne m'en fallut pas davantage, et en quelques instans, j'eus coupé toutes les paires que je voulais diviser. Comme dans les expériences précédentes, je ne fis la section que d'un seul côté, afin d'avoir un terme de comparaison. On conçoit avec quelle curiosité je suivis les effets de cette section, ils ne furent point douteux, le membre était complètement immobile et flasque, tandis qu'il con-

---

the blade of which, being very narrow, would permit of my cutting the roots, by pressing them with the sharp side of the instrument, against the posterior surface of the body of the vertebræ; but I was obliged to renounce this method on account of the large veins which the canal contains on that side, and which I opened at each progressive movement. In making these attempts, I perceived that by pulling the vertebral dura-mater, the anterior roots might be seen united in bundles, exactly where they pierce that membrane. I wanted nothing more, and in a few moments I had cut all the pairs which I wished to divide. As in the preceding experiments, I made the section on one side only, in order to have a point of comparison. It may be conceived with what curiosity I observed the effects of this section: they were not doubtful, the member was completely immovable and flaccid, at the same time preserving an

servait une sensibilité non équivoque. Enfin, pour ne rien négliger, j'ai coupé à la fois les racines antérieures et les postérieures; il y a eu perte absolue de sentiment et de mouvement.

J'ai répété et varié ces expériences sur plusieurs espèces d'animaux: les résultats que je viens d'énoncer se sont confirmés de la manière la plus complète, soit pour les membres antérieurs, soit pour les postérieurs. Je poursuis ces recherches, et j'en donnerai un récit plus détaillé dans le prochain numéro; IL ME SUFFIT DE POUVOIR AVANCER AUJOURD'HUI COMME POSITIF, QUE LES RACINES ANTÉRIEURES ET LES POSTÉRIEURES DES NERFS QUI NAISSENT À LA MOELLE ÉPINIÈRE, ONT DES FONCTIONS DIFFÉRENTES, QUE LES POSTÉRIEURES PARAISSENT PLUS PARTICULIÈREMENT DESTINÉES À LA SENSIBILITÉ, TANDIS QUE LES ANTÉRIEURES SEMBLENT PLUS SPÉCIALEMENT LIÉES AVEC LE MOUVEMENT.

---

unequivocal sensibility. Finally, that nothing might be neglected, I cut the anterior and posterior roots at the same time; there ensued absolute loss both of sensibility and of motion.

I have repeated and varied these experiments upon several species of animals: the results just announced were confirmed in the most complete manner, both for the posterior and anterior members. I am pursuing these researches, and I shall give a more detailed recital of them in the following number; IT IS SUFFICIENT FOR ME AT PRESENT TO BE ABLE TO ADVANCE AS POSITIVE, THAT THE ANTERIOR AND POSTERIOR ROOTS OF THE NERVES WHICH ARISE FROM THE SPINAL MARROW, HAVE DIFFERENT FUNCTIONS, THAT THE POSTERIOR APPEAR MORE PARTICULARLY DESTINED TO SENSIBILITY, WHILST THE ANTERIOR SEEM MORE ESPECIALLY ALLIED TO MOTION.

EXPÉRIENCES SUR LES FONCTIONS DES RACINES DES NERFS QUI NAISSENT DE LA MOËLLE ÉPINIÈRE.

PAR F. MAGENDIE.

Date of Publication—1822.

Journal de Physiologie Expérimentale et Pathologique.
4e Numéro. Octobre, 1822.

Les faits que j'ai annoncés dans le précédent numéro sont trop importans pour que je n'aie pas cherché à les éclairer par de nouvelles recherches.

J'ai d'abord voulu m'assurer si on ne pourrait pas couper les racines antérieures ou postérieures des nerfs spinaux sans ouvrir le grand canal de la dure-mère

---

EXPERIMENTS UPON THE FUNCTIONS OF THE ROOTS OF THE NERVES WHICH ARISE FROM THE SPINAL MARROW.

BY F. MAGENDIE.

Journal of Physiology Experimental and Pathological, No. IV. *October*, 1822.

The facts which I announced in the preceding number are too important to be passed over without my seeking to throw light upon them by new researches.

I at first wished to ascertain if it might not be possible to cut the anterior and posterior roots of the spinal nerves without opening the great canal of the vertebral dura-mater; because, by exposing the

vertébrale ; car, en exposant la moëlle épinière à l'air et à une température froide, on affaiblit sensiblement l'action nerveuse, et par suite on obtient d'une manière peu apparente les résultats que l'on cherche.

La disposition anatomique des parties ne rendait point la chose impossible ; car chaque faisceau de racine spinale chemine quelque temps dans un canal particulier, avant de se réunir et se confondre avec l'autre faisceau. En effet j'ai trouvé qu'à l'aide de ciseaux mousses par la pointe on peut enlever assez des lames et des parties latérales des vertèbres pour mettre à découvert le ganglion de chaque paire lombaire ; et alors avec un petit stylet on sépare sans trop de difficulté le canal qui contient les racines postérieures, et il n'y a plus de difficulté pour faire la section. Cette manière de faire l'expérience m'a donné les mêmes résultats que ceux que j'avais déjà observés; mais comme l'expérience est beaucoup plus

---

spinal marrow to the air and to a cold temperature, the nervous action is sensibly weakened, and consequently the results sought for are obtained in a manner but little apparent.

The anatomical position of the parts did not render the thing impossible ; for each bundle of spinal roots goes for some time in a particular canal before uniting and confounding itself with the other bundle. I found indeed that with the help of scissors blunt at the points, a sufficient quantity of the plates and lateral parts of the vertebræ may be taken away to expose the ganglion of each lumbar pair ; and then with a small stylet there is not much difficulty in separating the canal which contains the posterior roots, and the section becomes easy. This mode of making the experiment gave me the same results as those I had previously observed ; but as the experiment is much longer and more laborious than the preceding

longue et laborieuse qu'en suivant le procédé où l'on ouvre le grand canal de la dure-mère spinale, je ne crois pas qu'on doive suivre cette méthode de faire l'expérience de préférence à la première.

J'ai voulu ensuite soumettre à une épreuve particulière les résultats dont j'ai précédemment parlé. Chacun sait que la noix vomique détermine chez l'homme et les animaux des convulsions tétaniques générales très-violentes. Il était curieux de savoir si ces convulsions auraient encore lieu dans un membre dont les nerfs du mouvement seraient coupés, et si elles se montreraient aussi fortes qu'à l'ordinaire, la section des nerfs du sentiment étant faite. Le résultat a été tout-à-fait d'accord avec les précédens ; c'est-à-dire que sur un animal où les racines postérieures étaient coupées, le tétanos a été complet et aussi intense que si les racines spinales eussent été toutes intactes : au contraire, dans un animal où j'avais coupé les nerfs

---

one in which the great canal of the spinal dura-mater is opened, I do not think that this mode of making the experiment should be followed in preference to the first.

I afterwards wished to submit to more particular proof the results of which I have previously spoken. Every one knows that nux vomica determines both in man and animals, general and very violent tetanic convulsions. I was curious to ascertain if these convulsions would still take place in a member in which the nerves of motion had been cut, and if they would appear to be as strong as usual, a section of the nerves of sensation having been made. The result accorded entirely with the preceding; that is to say in an animal in which the posterior roots were cut, the tetanus was complete and as intense as if the spinal nerves had been untouched: on the contrary, in an animal in which I had cut the nerves of motion of

du mouvement de l'un des membres postérieurs, ce membre est resté souple et immobile dans le moment où, sous l'influence du poison, tous les autres muscles du corps éprouvaient les contractions tétaniques les plus prononcées.

En irritant directement les nerfs du sentiment, ou les racines spinales postérieures, produirait-on des contractions? Une irritation directe des nerfs du mouvement exciterait-elle de la douleur? Telles sont les questions que je me suis faites, et que l'expérience seule pouvait résoudre.

J'ai commencé par examiner sous ce rapport LES RACINES POSTÉRIEURES, ou les nerfs du sentiment. Voici ce que j'ai observé : *en pinçant, tiraillant, piquant ces racines, l'animal témoigne de la douleur;* MAIS ELLE N'EST POINT À COMPARER POUR L'INTENSITÉ AVEC CELLE QUI SE DÉVELOPPE SI L'ON TOUCHE, MÊME LÉGÈREMENT, LA MOELLE ÉPINIÈRE À L'EN-

---

one of the posterior members, the members remained supple and immovable at the time when, under the influence of the poison, all the other muscles of the body suffered the most violent tetanic convulsions.

On directly irritating the nerves of sensation, or the posterior spinal roots, would contractions be produced? Would a direct irritation of the nerves of motion excite pain? These were the questions which I asked myself and which experience alone could resolve.

With this view, I began to examine THE POSTERIOR ROOTS or the nerves of sensation. The following are the results of my observations : *in pinching, pulling, pricking these roots, the animal gives signs of pain;* BUT IT IS NOT TO BE COMPARED IN INTENSITY WITH THAT WHICH OCCURS IF THE SPINAL MARROW BE ONLY SLIGHTLY TOUCHED AT THE PART WHERE THESE ROOTS ARISE.

DROIT OÙ NAISSENT CES RACINES. *Presque toutes les fois que l'on excite ainsi les racines postérieures, il se produit des contractions dans les muscles où les nerfs se distribuent;* CES CONTRACTIONS SONT CEPENDANT PEU MARQUÉES, ET INFINIMENT PLUS FAIBLES QUE SI ON TOUCHE LA MOELLE ELLE-MÊME. QUAND ON COUPE A LA FOIS UN FAISCEAU DE RACINE POSTÉRIEURE, IL SE PRODUIT UN MOUVEMENT DE TOTALITÉ DANS LE MEMBRE OÙ LE FAISCEAU VA SE RENDRE.

J'ai répété les mêmes tentatives sur LES FAISCEAUX ANTÉRIEURS, et j'ai obtenu des résultats analogues, mais en sens inverse; car LES CONTRACTIONS *excitées par le pincement, la piqûre, etc., sont* TRÈS-FORTES ET MÊME CONVULSIVES, *tandis que les* SIGNES DE SENSIBILITÉ *sont* À PEINE VISIBLES. Ces faits sont donc confirmatifs de ceux que j'ai annoncés; seulement

---

Nearly every time that these posterior roots are thus excited, contractions are produced in the muscles to which the nerves are distributed; THESE CONTRACTIONS ARE HOWEVER BUT SLIGHTLY MARKED, AND INFINITELY WEAKER THAN IF THE SPINAL MARROW ITSELF BE TOUCHED. IF ONE OF THE POSTERIOR BUNDLES OF ROOTS BE CUT AT ONCE, A GENERAL MOVEMENT IS PRODUCED IN THE MEMBER TO WHICH THE BUNDLE GOES.

I have repeated the same experiments upon THE ANTERIOR BUNDLES, and I have obtained analogous results, but in an inverse sense; for THE CONTRACTIONS *excited by the pinching, pricking, &c. are* EXTREMELY STRONG AND EVEN CONVULSIVE, *whilst the* SIGNS OF SENSIBILITY *are* SCARCELY VISIBLE. These facts then are confirmative of those already announced; only they seem to

ils semblent établir que LE SENTIMENT N'EST PAS EXCLUSIVEMENT DANS LES RACINES POSTÉRIEURES, NON PLUS QUE LE MOUVEMENT DANS LES ANTÉRIEURES.

Cependant une difficulté pouvait s'élever. *Quand, dans les expériences qui précèdent, les racines ont été coupées, elles étaient continues avec la moëlle épinière ; l'ébranlement communiqué à celle-ci ne serait-il pas la véritable origine soit des contractions, soit de la douleur qu'ont éprouvée les animaux ? Pour lever ce doute,* J'AI REFAIT LES EXPÉRIENCES APRÈS AVOIR SÉPARÉ LES RACINES DE LA MOELLE ; ET JE DOIS DIRE QU'EXCEPTÉ SUR DEUX ANIMAUX, OÙ J'AI VU DES CONTRACTIONS QUAND JE PINÇAIS OU TIRAILLAIS LES FAISCEAUX ANTÉRIEURS ET POSTÉRIEURS, DANS TOUS LES AUTRES CAS JE N'AI OBSERVÉ AUCUN EFFET SENSIBLE DE L'IRRITATION DES RACINES ANTÉRIEURES OU POSTÉRIEURES AINSI SÉPARÉES DE LA MOELLE.

---

establish that SENSATION DOES NOT BELONG EXCLUSIVELY TO THE POSTERIOR ROOTS, ANY MORE THAN MOTION TO THE ANTERIOR.

Nevertheless a difficulty might arise. *When, in the preceding experiments, the roots were cut, they were continuous with the spinal marrow: might not the disturbance communicated to the latter have been the real origin, either of the contractions or of the pain felt by the animals? To remove this doubt,* I REPEATED THE EXPERIMENTS, AFTER HAVING SEPARATED THE ROOTS FROM THE SPINAL MARROW ; AND I OUGHT TO SAY THAT, WITH THE EXCEPTION OF TWO ANIMALS IN WHICH I SAW CONTRACTIONS UPON PINCHING AND PULLING THE ANTERIOR AND POSTERIOR BUNDLES, IN ALL THE REST I DID NOT OBSERVE ANY SENSIBLE EFFECT FROM THE IRRITATION OF THE ANTERIOR OR POSTERIOR ROOTS THUS SEPARATED FROM THE SPINAL MARROW.

J'avais encore *un autre genre d'épreuve à faire subir aux racines spinales ; c'était le galvanisme.* En conséquence j'ai excité ces parties par ce moyen, d'abord en les laissant dans leur état ordinaire, et ensuite en les coupant par leur extrémité spinale pour les placer sur un corps isolant. Dans ces divers cas J'AI OBTENU DES CONTRACTIONS AVEC LES DEUX SORTES DE RACINES ; mais les contractions qui suivaient l'excitation des racines antérieures étaient en général bien plus fortes et bien plus complètes que celles qui naissaient quand le courant électrique s'établissait par les postérieures. Les mêmes phénomènes avaient lieu soit qu'on appliquât le pole zinc ou le pole cuivre sur le nerf.

Il me reste maintenant à rendre compte des recherches que j'ai faites pour tâcher de suivre le sentiment et le mouvement isolés au-delà des racines des nerfs, c'est-à-dire dans la moëlle épinière ; je m'en occuperai incessamment.

I had still to make *another kind of experiment on the spinal roots ; that of galvanism.* By its means, I accordingly excited these parts, first leaving them in their ordinary state, and afterwards cutting them at their spinal extremities to place them upon an isolating body. In these various cases, I OBTAINED CONTRACTIONS FROM EACH SORT OF ROOTS ; but those which followed the excitation of the anterior roots were in general much stronger and more complete than those which took place when the electric current operated upon the posterior. The same phenomena took place either by applying the zinc or copper pole to the nerve.

It now remains for me to give an account of my researches to endeavour to follow motion and sensation distinctly beyond the roots of the nerves, that is to say, into the spinal marrow ; this is the subject of my present occupation.

Avant de terminer cet article, je dois donner quelques éclaircissemens sur la nouveauté des résultats que j'ai annoncés.

Quand j'ai écrit la note contenue dans le numéro précédent, je croyais être le premier qui eût songé à couper les racines des nerfs spinaux ; mais je fus bientôt détrompé par un petit écrit de M. Schaw, que ce jeune et laborieux médecin eut la complaisance de m'envoyer dès qu'il eut reçu le numéro de mon journal. Il est dit dans cet écrit que M. Ch. Bell avait fait cette section *il y a treize ans*,* et qu'il avait reconnu que la section des racines postérieures n'empêchait pas les mouvemens de continuer. M. Schaw ajoute que M. Ch. Bell avait consigné ce résultat dans une

---

Before finishing this article, I ought to give some further explanations as to the novelty of the results which I have announced.

When I wrote the note contained in the preceding number, I believed I was the first who had thought of dividing the roots of the spinal nerves; but I was soon undeceived by a small work by Mr. Shaw, which this young and laborious practitioner had the politeness to send me as soon as he had received the number of my journal. It is said in that work that Mr. Charles Bell made this section *thirteen years ago*, and that he had discovered that the section of the posterior roots did not prevent the continuance of motion. Mr. Shaw adds that Mr. Charles Bell had stated this result in a small

---

* Thirteen years before 1822, the date of this Paper, would make the date of printing the "Idea of a NEW ANATOMY OF THE BRAIN," 1809—*just as early* as Mr. Walker's "NEW ANATOMY AND PHYSIOLOGY OF THE BRAIN! yet Sir C. Bell now states that his NEW ANATOMY was really two years later than Mr. Walker's NEW ANATOMY! The coincidence in the two Titles is certainly strange.

petite brochure imprimée seulement pour ses amis, mais non pour la publication. J'ai aussitôt demandé à M. Schaw qu'il voulût bien m'envoyer, s'il était possible, la brochure de M. Ch. Bell, afin que je lui rendisse toute la justice qui lui serait due. Peu de jours après je l'ai reçue de M. Schaw.

Cette brochure a pour titre :

Idea of a NEW ANATOMY OF THE BRAIN, *submitted for the Observations of his Friends, by* CH. BELL, F.R.S.E. Elle est très-curieuse en ce qu'on y remarque le germe des récentes découvertes de l'auteur sur le système nerveux. A la page 22 on trouve le passage indiqué par Schaw ; je le transcris en entier :

" Next considering that the spinal nerves have a double root, and being of opinion that the properties of the nerves are derived from their connections with the parts of the brain, I thought that I had an opportunity of putting my opinion to the test of experiment, and of proving at the same time that nerves of

---

pamphlet printed solely for the use of his friends, but not for publication. I immediately asked Mr. Shaw to have the kindness to send me if possible the pamphlet of Mr. Charles Bell, in order that I might render him all the justice that was his due. A few days afterwards I received it from Mr. Shaw.

This pamphlet is entitled :

Idea of a NEW ANATOMY OF THE BRAIN, *submitted for the Observations of his Friends, by* CHARLES BELL, F.R.S.E. It is very curious, inasmuch as there is to be found in it the germ of the recent discoveries of the author in the nervous system. At page 22, the passage indicated by Shaw is to be found : I shall transcribe the whole of it.

(As given in the text.)

different endowments were in the same cord and held by the same sheath.

" On laying bare the roots of the spinal nerves, I found that I could cut across the fasciculus of nerves, which took its origin from the posterior portion of the spinal marrow, without convulsing the muscles of the back; but that on touching the anterior fasciculus with the point of a knife, the muscles of the back were immediately convulsed."

On voit par cette citation d'un ouvrage que je ne pouvais connaître, puisqu'il n'a point été publié, que *M. Bell, conduit par ses ingénieuses idées sur le système nerveux, a été bien près de découvrir les fonctions des racines spinales;* TOUTEFOIS LE FAIT QUE LES ANTÉRIEURES SONT DESTINÉES AU MOUVEMENT, TANDIS QUE LES POSTÉRIEURES APPARTIENNENT PLUS PARTICULIÈREMENT AU SENTIMENT, PARAIT LUI AVOIR ÉCHAPPÉ: C'EST DONC À AVOIR ÉTABLI CE FAIT D'UNE MANIÈRE POSITIVE QUE JE DOIS BORNER MES PRÉTENTIONS.

It is seen by this citation of a work which I could not know, since it had not been published, that *Mr. Bell, conducted by his ingenious ideas on the nervous system, was very near discovering the functions of the spinal roots;* AT THE SAME TIME, THE FACT THAT THE ANTERIOR ARE DESTINED TO MOTION, WHILST THE POSTERIOR BELONG MORE ESPECIALLY TO SENSATION, APPEARS TO HAVE ESCAPED HIM: IT IS THEN TO THE ESTABLISHMENT OF THIS FACT IN A POSITIVE MANNER THAT I MUST LIMIT MY PRETENSIONS.

NOTE SUR LE SIÈGE DU MOUVEMENT ET SENTIMENT DANS LA MOËLLE ÉPINIÈRE.

PAR F. MAGENDIE.

Date of Publication—1823.

Journal de Physiologie Expérimentale et Pathologique. *Année* 1823.

LES expériences que j'ai publiées sur les fonctions des racines des nerfs spinaux, et qui montrent que les antérieures sont destinées au mouvement, tandis que les postérieures appartiennent au sentiment, conduisaient naturellement à examiner si les côtés antérieurs et postérieurs de la moëlle épinière ne seraient point en rapport de propriétés avec les filets nerveux. Le fait confirme ici la conjecture : *si on met à nu la moëlle*

NOTE ON THE SEAT OF MOTION AND SENSATION IN THE SPINAL MARROW,

BY F. MAGENDIE.

Journal of Experimental and Pathological Physiology, 1823.

THE experiments which I have published on the functions of the roots of the spinal nerves, and which show that the anterior are destined to motion, whilst the posterior belong to sensation, naturally led me to examine if the anterior and posterior sides of the spinal marrow had not similar properties with the nervous filaments. Fact here confirms conjecture: *If the spinal marrow is exposed at any*

dans un point quelconque de sa longueur, et si on la touche ou la pique doucement en arrière, sur les deux cordons placés entre les racines postérieures, l'animal donne des signes d'une exquise sensibilité ; si, au contraire, on fait les mêmes tentatives sur la partie antérieure, les indices de sensibilité sont à peine visibles. Il en est de même de la partie centrale de la moëlle. On peut la toucher, la déchirer pour ainsi dire impunément, en prenant toutefois les précautions nécessaires afin d'éviter la substance médullaire circonvoisine. J'ai plusieurs fois enfoncé des stylets dans presque toute la longueur de la moëlle, sans que le mouvement ni la sensibilité de l'animal me parussent diminués.

En général, les propriétés de la moëlle spinale paraissent résider à la surface de cette partie, cela est du moins évident quant à la sensibilité. *Pour peu que l'on touche aux cordons postérieurs même revêtus de leurs membranes vasculaires, on obtient des signes d'une*

---

point of its length, and if touched or pricked gently behind, upon the two cords placed between the posterior roots, the animal exhibits signs of the most exquisite sensibility ; if, on the contrary, the same attempts are made on the anterior part, the indications of sensibility are scarcely visible. It is the same with the central part of the spinal marrow. It may be touched, torn even we may say, with impunity, always taking the precaution necessary to avoid touching the surrounding medullary substance. I have several times plunged stylets through almost the whole length of the spinal marrow, without either the motions or the sensibility of the animal appearing to be diminished.

In general, the properties of the spinal marrow appear to reside on the surface of that part; this is at least evident with respect to sensibility. *The slightest touch of the posterior cords even when enclosed in their vascular membranes, causes signs of intense pain, and,* WHAT

vive douleur, et, CE QUI EST DIGNE DE REMARQUE, DES CONTRACTIONS TRÈS-PRONONCÉES DANS LES MUSCLES QUI REÇOIVENT LEURS NERFS INFÉRIEUREMENT À L'ENDROIT TOUCHÉ. Les contractions ne se montrent que du côté du cordon que l'on irrite.

Il serait sans doute bien à désirer qu'on pût savoir comment le sentiment et le mouvement se propagent de la moëlle dans le cerveau. LA DISPOSITION ANATOMIQUE INDIQUE QUE LE SENTIMENT DOIT SE DIRIGER PLUS PARTICULIÈRMENT VERS LE CERVELET, ET LE MOUVEMENT VERS LE CERVEAU : mais l'anatomie ne suffit pas ; il faut que *la physiologie* et *les faits pathologiques* viennent confirmer l'indication ; or jusqu'ici *ni l'un ni l'autre de ces moyens n'a établi ce que l'anatomie semble montrer* d'une manière si évidente. (1) LES LÉSIONS

(1) Du moins si on s'en rapporte aux descriptions données par les auteurs les plus récents. Il me semble cependant qu'on pourrait

---

IS WORTHY OF REMARK, VERY MARKED CONTRACTIONS IN THE MUSCLES RECEIVING THEIR NERVES FROM BELOW THE PART TOUCHED. The contractions show themselves only on the same side with the cord which receives the irritation.

It would, without doubt, be very desirable to know how sensation and motion are propagated from the spinal marrow to the brain. THE ANATOMICAL STRUCTURE INDICATES THAT SENSATION OUGHT TO BE DIRECTED MORE PARTICULARLY TO THE CEREBELLUM, AND MOTION TO THE CEREBRUM: but anatomy does not suffice; it is necessary that *physiology* and *pathological facts* should confirm the indication; and hitherto *neither one nor the other of these means have established what anatomy seems to show* in so evident a manner.* LESIONS OF THE CEREBELLUM DO NOT

* At least if we refer to the descriptions given by the most recent authors. It seems to me, however, that some facts might be added

DU CERVELET NE FONT POINT PERDRE LA SENSIBILITÉ. LA SOUSTRACTION DES HÉMISPHÈRES N'EMPORTE PAS NÉCESSAIREMENT LA PERTE DU MOUVEMENT; l'assertion contraire, annoncée par M. Rolando, n'est point exacte; ce médecin me paraît s'être laissé tromper par une circonstance accidentelle. Quand on enlève les hémisphères en totalité, il se fait aussitôt un épanchement sanguin, et il se forme un caillot qui remplit la cavité du crâne, comprime la moëlle allongée, et produit l'état d'assoupissement observé par M. Rolando. Mais si on empêche la formation de ce caillot, les symptômes sont tout différens; les animaux sont dans une agitation continuelle; ils

ajouter quelques faits à l'histoire anatomique de la jonction de la moëlle avec le cerveau et le cervelet. J'ai commencé des recherches sur ce point, devenu aujourd'hui plus important qu'il n'était naguères.

CAUSE LOSS OF SENSIBILITY. THE SUBTRACTION OF THE HEMISPHERES DOES NOT NECESSARILY CAUSE THE LOSS OF MOTION: the contrary assertion, announced by M. Rolando, is not exact; it appears to me that this physician has allowed himself to be deceived by an accidental circumstance. When the whole of the hemispheres are taken away, an effusion of blood immediately takes place, and a clot forms which fills the cavity of the skull, compresses the medulla oblongata, and produces the state of lethargy observed by M. Rolando. But if this clot of blood be prevented from forming, the symptoms are entirely different: the animals are in continual

to the anatomical description of the junction of the spinal marrow with the cerebrum and cerebellum. I have commenced some researches upon this point, now become of much more importance than formerly.

courent ou volent avec une agilité singulière, à moins qu'ils ne soient trop affaiblis par la perte du sang. Les animaux sur laquelle cette expérience réussit le mieux, sont des petits lapins d'un mois ou six semaines, et de jeunes geais et des pies qui commencent à manger seuls. Il est curieux de les voir spontanément courir, sauter, etc., après la soustraction complète de toutes les parties du cerveau placées un peu au-devant des tubercules optiques. (1)

Mais si la section est faite immédiatement au-devant de ces dernières éminences, tout s'arrête ; l'animal tombe sur le côté, la tête renversée en arrière, les pattes entièrement roides et dirigées en avant.

(1) Les chats nouveau-nés n'ont que des mouvements incertains et généralement assez lents : ces animaux tournent sur eux-mêmes en divers sens. La soustraction des hémisphères leur donne ordinairement la faculté de marcher en avant avec une agilité et une activité singulières.

---

agitation ; they run or fly with singular agility, unless indeed they are too much weakened by the loss of blood. The animals upon which this experiment succeeds best, are small rabbits of the age of about a month or six weeks, and young jays or magpies just beginning to feed themselves. It is curious to see them run spontaneously, leap, &c., after the complete subtraction of all the parts of the cerebrum, placed a little before the optic tubercles.*

But if the section be made immediately before these last eminences, all is stopped ; the animal falls upon its side, the head thrown back, the paws quite rigid and thrown forward. I have seen young

* Young kittens display movements which are uncertain and in general rather slow : these animals turn round in divers ways. The subtraction of the hemispheres generally gives them the faculty of moving forwards with singular activity and agility.

J'ai vu de jeunes lapins rester plusieurs heures dans cette position. Pour la faire cesser, il suffit de faire une section derrière les tubercules optiques. Aussitôt les pattes antérieures perdent leur roideur, et le plus souvent se fléchissent ainsi que les postérieures, et la tête est ramenée en avant. Il me paraît évident, d'après ces faits, que les couches optiques, les cuisses du cerveau, les tubercules quadrijumeaux, ont des fonctions relatives aux mouvements, et que ces parties ont besoin d'être examinées sous ce nouveau point de vue.

Les effets de la soustraction partielle ou totale du cervelet sont bien plus difficiles à observer, à raison de l'hémorragie considérable qui accompagne toujours la blessure de cet organe, des épanchemens qui en sont la suite inévitable, et de la compression de la moëlle épinière. Je n'ai pas encore pu assigner à chacun de ces effets la part qu'il prend dans les phénomènes

---

rabbits remain for several hours in this position. To cause its cessation, it suffices to make a section behind the optic tubercles. Immediately the anterior paws lose their rigidity, and generally bend, as well as the posterior ones, and the head is again brought forward. It appears evident to me, from these facts, that the thalami, the crura of the cerebrum, the corpora quadrigemina, have functions relative to motion, and that these parts require to be examined in this new point of view.

The effects of the partial or total subtraction of the cerebellum are much more difficult to be observed, on account of the considerable hemorrhage which always accompanies a wound of this organ, the effusions of blood which are the inevitable consequence, and the compression of the spinal marrow. I have not yet been able to assign to each of these effects the part it takes in the phenomena which

qui se produisent lors des blessures ou des ablations du cervelet; mais *il est pourtant facile de constater que des lésions profondes du cervelet et des ablations totales ne font pas perdre la sensibilité.* Les expériences de Lorry, de Legallois, etc., ont d'ailleurs démontré que cette propriété est inhérente à la moëlle spinale. Il faut espérer que cette difficulté sera bientôt levée, car plusieurs personnes très-zélées s'occupent de recherches sur ce point, et moi-même je fais tous mes efforts pour arriver à quelque chose de satisfaisant sur cette importante question.

Ce que j'ai remarqué jusqu'ici de plus constant, c'est que *le cervelet semble nécessaire à l'intégrité des mouvemens en avant.* Toute blessure un peu grave du cervelet rend toute progression en avant impossible, et développe le plus souvent, au contraire, un ensemble de mouvemens qui se rapportent à l'action de reculer. Un canard, auquel j'avais enlevé une grande

---

are produced by wounds or ablation of the cerebellum; *nevertheless it is easy to prove that deep lesions and total ablations of the cerebellum do not cause a loss of sensibility.* The experiments of Lorry, Legallois, &c. have besides shown that this property is inherent in the spinal marrow. It is to be hoped that this difficulty will soon be obviated, as several very zealous persons are occupied in researches on this point, and I myself make every effort to arrive at some satisfactory conclusion upon this important question.

What I have hitherto remarked as most certain, is, that *the cerebellum appears necessary to the integrity of movements forward.* Every wound of any importance of the cerebellum renders all progression forward impossible, and generally developes, on the contrary, an assemblage of movements which relate to the act of going backward. A duck, from which I had removed a great part of the

partie du cervelet, ne nageait plus qu'en reculant, et il n'a plus fait d'autre mouvement progressif durant huit jours.

En attendant des recherches ultérieures, voici un fait de la plus haute importance touchant les fonctions des faisceaux antérieurs et postérieurs de la moëlle épinière, et qui vient confirmer ce que j'ai avancé sur les usages de ces parties. Je le dois à la complaisance de M. le professeur Royer-Collard.

Altération de la partie antérieure de la moëlle épinière, observée à la maison de santé de Charenton, par M. Royer-Collard.

[In this case, the patient's gait was reeling, his lower extremities tottering, and the upper extremities free. The lower extremities becoming more and more feeble, the patient was unable to walk, and he remained for about seven years with the thighs bent on the pelvis, and the legs on the thighs, without performing any motion by means of these parts, which, nevertheless, preserved sensibility. After death, while the posterior part of the spinal marrow was sound, its anterior part, as far as the anterior roots of

---

cerebellum, swam in no other direction than backward, and for eight days made no other movement.

Whilst waiting for ulterior researches, the following is a fact of the highest importance touching the functions of the anterior and posterior bundles of the spinal marrow, and which confirms what I have advanced as to the use of these parts. I owe it to the politeness of M. Professor Royer-Collard.

Alteration of the anterior part of the spinal marrow observed in the establishment for health at Charenton, by M. Royer-Collard.

(See the text.)

the spinal nerves, as well as the olivary and pyramidal bodies were softened, and this state extended to the pons Varolii, the crura cerebri, the thalami, the striated bodies, and some of the cerebral convolutions, especially about the middle of the right lobe.]

Cette observation n'est-elle pas propre à mettre dans leur jour les propriétés distinctes de la partie antérieure et de la partie postérieure de la moëlle? Cependant *il faut dire que les mouvemens des bras étaient en partie conservés ;* le rédacteur de la note ne le dit pas, mais M. Royer-Collard me l'a assuré verbalement. Or, *cette dernière circonstance fait sentir la nécessité d'un nouvel examen et de l'anatomie de la moëlle et de ses phénomènes vitaux.* Cette partie est beacoup plus compliquée à sa région supérieure que partout ailleurs, et nous ne savons rien encore des usages des corps olivaires, des pyramides antérieures et postérieures, etc.

Je fais en ce moment des recherches sur ces divers points.

Is not this case calculated to throw light upon the distinct properties of the anterior aud posterior parts of the spinal marrow? Nevertheless, *we must say that the motion of the arms was in part preserved;* the person who drew up the note does not say so, but M. Royer-Collard assured me of it verbally. Now, *this last circumstance shows the necessity of a new examination, both of the anatomy of the spinal marrow and of its vital phenomena.* This part is much more complicated in its superior region than any where else, and we know as yet nothing of the functions of the olivary bodies, of the anterior and posterior pyramids, &c.

I am at the present moment occupied in researches upon these different points.

NOTE BY THE EDITOR.

Thus concludes this first series of papers—those relative to the nervous system generally. In an enlarged view of these, it is remarkable that the last, or those of Magendie, tend toward a view, the opposite of the first, or those of Walker. Still, however, Magendie allows both sensation and motion to anterior as well as to posterior parts. Muller's experiments on frogs would, indeed, indicate a distinct appropriation of these organs and functions respectively : but the anomalous organization of these animals, lately discovered by Volkman, the absence of any decided distinction in animals below these—turtles and rays, discovered by Hall, and the doubt as to whether, as mentioned in the Introductory Remarks, all experiments have not hitherto been made on mere vital or ganglionic fibrils instead of mental nerves, spinal columns and cerebral masses, will probably appear, to all who are not partizans, as calculated to leave the great question still *sub judice.*

DOCUMENTS RELATIVE TO THE SPINAL MARROW, ETC.

SENSATION THE CAUSE OF A CONSERVATIVE MOTION IN THE WHOLE OR IN THE SEPARATED PARTS OF ANIMALS—INVOLUNTARY MOTION; THE CENTRE OF THIS BEING THE BRAIN OR SPINAL MARROW.

BY ROBERT WHYTT, M.D.

Date of Publication — 1751.

From an Essay on the Vital and Involuntary Motions of Animals, Works, Edit. 1768, *pages,* 152, 162, 203, &c.

BY means of *this connecting medium* (THE SENTIENT PRINCIPLE), the various impressions made on the several parts of the body, either by external or internal causes, are transmitted, and perceived by the mind; in consequence of which it may determine the nervous influence variously into the different organs, and so become the cause of all the VITAL AND INVOLUNTARY MOTIONS, as well as of the ANIMAL AND VOLUNTARY. *It seems to act necessarily, and as a sentient principle only, when its power is exerted in causing the* FORMER; but, *in producing the* LATTER, *it acts freely, and both as a sentient and rational agent.*—p. 152.

The *motions performed* by us *in consequence of irritation,* are owing to the original constitution of our frame, whence the soul or *sentient principle,* immediately, and *without any previous ratiocination,* endeavours by all means, and in the most effectual manner, to avoid or *get rid of every disagreeable sensation* conveyed to it by *whatever hurts or annoys the body.*—p. 162.

Not to perplex ourselves with metaphysical difficulties, we shall recite A FEW EXPERIMENTS AND OBSERVATIONS, FROM WHICH WE ARE LED, BY ANALOGY, TO CONCLUDE THAT THE MOTIONS OF THE SEPARATED PARTS OF ANIMALS ARE OWING TO THE SOUL OR SENTIENT PRINCIPLE STILL CONTINUING TO ACT IN THEM.

A frog lives, and moves its members, for half an hour after its head is cut off; nay, when the body of a frog is divided into two, both the anterior and posterior extremities preserve life and a power of motion for a considerable time.

A young cock, whose head Dr. Kaau suddenly cut off with a sharp razor, as he was running with great eagerness to his food, went on in a straight line 23 Rhinland feet, and would have gone farther had he not met with an obstacle which stopped him. The story, therefore, mentioned by Lord Verulam, of an ostrich running along the stage after its head was struck off with a forked arrow by one of the Roman emperors, is not improbable.

A viper, after being deprived of its head and entrails, moved towards a heap of stones in a garden where it used to hide itself.

The bodies of vipers not only move two or three days after they have been deprived of their skin, head, heart, and other bowels, but are also manifestly sensible of punctures by means of which they may be made to move with greater vivacity.

The female butterflies into which silk worms have been metamorphosed, not only admit the male, after losing their heads, but also lay eggs.

Redi informs us, that a land-tortoise, whose brain he extracted by a hole in its scull, in the beginning of November, lived to the middle of May following. Immediately after the loss of its brain, it shut its eyes, nor ever opened them any more, but continued to move and walk about until the time of its death. When the skull was opened, its cavity appeared clean and smooth, and nothing was found in it except a small dry clot of blood. The same experiment he repeated on various other tortoises, some of which lived a longer, others a shorter time, but none of them less than fifty days.

A large tortoise, whose head Redi cut off, allowing the blood to flow freely from the open vessels of its neck, lived twenty-three days; and though it did not walk about like those which were deprived of their brain, yet as often as its fore or hind feet were pricked, it moved them with force, and was convulsed. In two tortoises which he opened fifteen days after decollation, he saw the heart beating as in a living animal, and the blood circulating through it.

Here, we are naturally led to observe, that while those animals who have a small *brain* and large *spinal marrow*, live long after decollation, man, and most quadrupeds, which have a large brain, survive the loss of it only for a few moments.

If the motions of a tortoise after decollation, or the loss of its brain, cannot proceed from mere mechanism, but must be undoubtedly ascribed to the living principle which was the cause of its motions in a sound state; and, if the same is true of the actions performed by butterflies after the loss of their heads, it must follow, that the motions and other signs of life which are observed in the body and limbs of a frog for above half an hour after its head is cut off, are to be attributed to the sentient principle, to which its motions and actions were owing when in an entire state; and if so, then the motions of this body, when divided into two parts, must also be referred to the same cause, since they are of a like kind, although of shorter duration. Shall we then deny that the motions of its separated heart and limbs, which are similar to these, and are increased and renewed by the application of the same causes, proceed from the sentient principle still acting in these parts?

This would be to neglect the strongest analogy; and we should be the more inexcusable, as no other cause has hitherto been assigned, so well accounting for these appearances.

We have no other way to satisfy ourselves that an animal is alive, or endued with feeling, but by observing, whether it shews an uneasiness when any thing hurts, or tends to destroy any of its parts, and an endeavour to remove or avoid it. Since, therefore, the bodies of vipers make just the same kind of motions when pricked with a sharp instrument, two or three days after losing their head, heart, and other *viscera*, as if they were entire, we are naturally led to conclude, that they are still, in some sense, alive and endued with feeling, i. e. animated by a sentient principle. And as the muscular parts of these creatures move after being cut in pieces, and are sensible of punctures, it also follows, that they continue still to be animated.*

* *Since the nerves, which are continuations of the medullary substance of the brain and spinal marrow, have been proved to retain their powers of feeling, and of putting the muscles in motion for some time after their connection with the brain is cut off, we have reason to believe that the motions excited by stimuli in the muscles of animals, after they are separated from their bodies, are owing to some kind of feeling or simple sensation* (such as oysters and other animals of the lowest class, who have no brain, are endued with) *in those muscles or their nerves, which, though not attended with any reflex* CONSCIOUSNESS, *a power the soul only exercises in the* BRAIN, *is nevertheless the immediate occasion of all those motions which arise from the irritation of the fibres of the muscles, whether they be con-*

Lastly, if the motions of the muscles in the limbs of a cock, after decollation, are, without dispute, owing to its soul; may we not also ascribe to the same principle the like, but less remarkable motions in men and quadrupeds, after their heads are struck off; and, consequently, the tremulous motions and palpitations of their hearts too, after death or separation from their bodies?

To sum up all in a few words; from what has been said, it appears evident that THE INVOLUNTARY MOTIONS OF LIVING ANIMALS, AND THE ALTERNATE CONTRACTIONS OF THEIR MUSCLES, AFTER THE GENERAL DEATH OF THE BODY, OR THEIR BEING SEPARATED FROM IT, ARE OWING TO ONE AND THE SAME CAUSE, VIZ. AN IRRITATION OF THEIR FIBRES OR NERVES, or of such parts as are nearly connected with them. *If then, if as we have shewn* (Sect. x.) *that the motions of animal fibres, from a stimulus, most certainly bespeaks a* FEELING, *and cannot be explained unless we admit it; and if feeling be not a property of*

nected with the other parts of the body, or newly separated from them.

And here it is proper to remark, that while those motions which are occasioned by stimulating the fibres of any muscle, continue for some little time after its communication with the brain, by means of the nerves, has been cut off; *such motions as proceed from sympathy, and are owing to the irritation of some distant part, cease as soon as the* BRAIN *is rendered unfit for action, or the communication with it interrupted, because they depend on a* PERCEPTION *in that organ from which the nerves proceed, and where alone the cause of their sympathy is to be found.*

matter, but owing to a superior principle, it must follow, that THE MOTIONS OF THE HEART, AND OTHER MUSCLES OF ANIMALS, AFTER BEING SEPARATED FROM THEIR BODIES, ARE TO BE ASCRIBED TO THIS PRINCIPLE; and that any difficulties which may appear in this matter are owing to our ignorance of the nature of the soul, of the manner of its existence, &c.

From his Observations on Sensibility and Irritability; Works, Edit. 1768, *page* 287, *et seq.*

It will be objected: How can there be any sensibility of feeling in a nerve whose communication with the brain is cut off?——In answer to which, it may be said, that, since we have good reasons for believing that the parts of many insects continue to be sensible for a considerable time after they have been divided from each other; and that the bodies of some larger animals continue to live and feel after they are deprived of their heads: Why may we not suppose that the muscles of men preserve some degree of sensibility for a few moments after their nerves are tied or cut; although we may not be able to account for this from any thing we know of the nature of the body, or of the manner in which the soul is present with, or acts upon it.*

* Why may not a muscle, whose nerve is tied or cut, continue for some little time, sensible and irritable? *Its sensibility will not indeed be attended with what is called* CONSCIOUSNESS, *as distin-*

Redi informs us that the head of a viper will bite half an hour after it is cut off from the body, (*Vid. Jacobæi Observat. de Ranis et Lacert. p.* 58); and I have often observed, that the head of a frog, after being separated from the body, not only continued, for above half an hour, to move the eyelids, nostrils and muscles of the lower jaw, when the brain or the skin of the head was touched with a probe, but sometimes moved the eyes and eye-lids, when nothing touched it, and as it were of its own accord; so that, without too much scepticism, we cannot deny that the head continues to be animated for some time

guished from simple sensation; because this reflex act, by which a person knows his thoughts or sensations to be his own, is a faculty of the soul exercised in the BRAIN *only,* with which all communication is now cut off.

The more probable opinion seems to be, that *the soul is equally present in the extremities of the nerves through the whole body as in the brain. In those, it is only capable of feeling or simple sensation; but in this, it exercises the powers of reflex consciousness and reason. When the communication of any part with the brain is cut off, the simple sensation of feeling excited in such part is no longer perceived by the soul in the brain; and therefore is not attended with reflex consciousness:* the nerves being then also separated from the brain, soon become unfit to perform their functions; hence the powers of simple sensation and motion in the part, if it be muscular, cease by degrees, till at last it becomes quite dead. The communication, therefore, between the several organs and the brain, is not only necessary to preserve their nerves, by means of some influence transmitted to them in due order for performing their functions and being properly affected by their several objects, but also, that the soul, as a conscious and rational being, may be acquainted with these impressions.

after it is separated from the body, and to perform not only involuntary motions when stimulated, but, *in appearance*, also voluntary ones. In like manner, the body of a frog, after being divided from the head, preserves the power of motion for above an hour; and when its hind feet or toes are cut, or otherwise hurt, the muscles of its thighs, legs and trunk are strongly contracted, by which it raises its body from the table, and sometimes moves from one place to another. When the muscles of the thighs are pricked or cut with a knife, they are excited into contraction; but neither they, nor the neighbouring muscles, are near so strongly convulsed as when the toes are wounded. Whence should this happen; and *why should not the muscles of the legs and thighs be more strongly convulsed, when they themselves are wounded, than when the toes are treated in the same manner?* This would be the case, if the motions of irritated muscles were owing to some property of the insensible matter composing them. But, *if, as we imagine, they are all to be derived from feeling, it is easy to see, that, as the feet and toes are more sensible of pain when wounded, than the muscles of the legs or thighs, stronger convulsions must be occasioned by an irritation of the former than of the latter.*

If the soul were confined to the brain, as many have believed, whence is it that a pigeon not only lives for several hours after being deprived of its brain, but also flies from one place to another? And to what cause are we to ascribe the continuance of life and motion in a viper for three days after its head is cut off, and in a tortoise for three weeks after decollation, and six months after the loss of its brain? The motions performed by these animals cannot surely be attributed to their material part alone; unless we shall deny them a soul altogether, and, with Des Cartes, refer all their actions to their corporeal machinery. The late reverend and learned Dr. Hales informed me, that *having many years since tied a ligature about the neck of a frog to prevent any effusion of blood, he cut off its head, and, thirty hours after, observed the blood circulating freely in the web of the foot: the frog also at this time moved its body when stimulated: but that,* ON THRUSTING A NEEDLE DOWN THE SPINAL MARROW, THE ANIMAL WAS STRONGLY CONVULSED, AND IMMEDIATELY AFTER BECAME MOTIONLESS.

In his paper "On the Sympathy of the Nerves," Works, page 510, *Whytt adds:*

——When the nerve going to any muscle is irritated, there is no motion excited in any part, except in the muscle to which it is distributed. Does it not hence appear highly probable, that THE VARIOUS SYMPATHETIC MOTIONS OF ANIMALS PRODUCED BY IRRITATION, WHETHER IN A SOUND OR MORBID STATE, ARE OWING, NOT TO ANY UNION OR CONNECTION OF THEIR NERVES, BUT TO PARTICULAR SENSATIONS EXCITED IN CERTAIN ORGANS, AND THENCE COMMU-

NICATED TO THE BRAIN OR SPINAL MARROW? For, if this were not the case, why should not the diaphragm, for example, be convulsed, by irritating the nerves that go to the bladder and intestinum rectum, as well as when these parts themselves are affected by an unusual stimulus?

INVOLUNTARY MOTIONS REFLECTED FROM THE SENSORIUM COMMUNE.

BY GEORGIUS PROCHASKA,

PROFESSOR OF ANATOMY, ETC.

Date of Publication—1784.

From Commentatio de Functionibus Systematis Nervosi, Opera Minora, Edit. 1800, *Vol. II. page* 150 *et seq.*

QUID sensorium commune, quæ ejus munia, et quæ sedes?

IMPRESSIONES EXTERNÆ, QUÆ IN NERVOS SENSORIOS FIUNT, PER TOTAM EORUM LONGITUDINEM CELERRIME AD ORIGINEM USQUE PROPAGANTUR; QUO UBI PERVENERUNT, REFLECTUNTUR CERTA LEGE, ET IN CERTOS AC RESPONDENTES NERVOS MOTORIOS TRANSEUNT, PER QUOS ITERUM CELERRIME USQUE AD MUSCULOS PROPAGATÆ MOTUS CERTOS AC DETERMINATOS EXCITANT. Hic locus, in quo tanquam centro nervi tam sensui quam motui dicati concurrunt, ac communicant, et

---

What are the Sensorium Commune, its functions, and its seat?

EXTERNAL IMPRESSIONS, WHICH ARE MADE UPON THE SENSORIAL NERVES, ARE PROPAGATED RAPIDLY THROUGH THEIR WHOLE LENGTH TO THEIR ORIGIN; WHERE, WHEN THEY HAVE ARRIVED, THEY ARE REFLECTED ACCORDING TO A CERTAIN LAW, AND PASS INTO CERTAIN AND CORRESPONDING MOTOR NERVES, THROUGH WHICH, AGAIN RAPIDLY PROPAGATED EVEN TO THE MUSCLES, THEY EXCITE CERTAIN AND DETERMINATE MOTIONS. This place, in which, as in a centre, the nerves appropriated to sense as well as motion, meet and communicate, and in

in quo impressiones nervorum sensoriorum reflectuntur in nervos motorios, vocatur, termino plerisque Physiologis jam recepto, *sensorium commune.*

Totum cerebrum cerebellumque certe non videtur ad sensorium commune constituendum spectare, quæ partes systematis nervosi videntur potius instrumenta esse, quibus anima immediate utitur, ad actiones suas, animales dictas, peragendas; sed sensorium commune proprie dictum se per medullam oblongatam, crura cerebri cerebellique; etiam thalamorum opticorum partem, et totam medullam spinalem, verbo, quam late patet nervorum origo, extendere non improbabile utique videtur. Ad medullam spinalem usque sensorium commune extendi docent motus in animalibus decapitatis superstites, qui sine nervorum ex medulla spinali oriundorum consensu ac commercio fieri non possent; nam rana decapitata si pungitur, non tantum punctam partem

---

which the impressions of the sensorial nerves are reflected upon the motor nerves, is called the Sensorium Commune—a term already received by most physiologists.

The whole cerebrum and cerebellum certainly do not seem to belong to the composition of the sensorium commune: these parts of the nervous system appear to be rather the instruments which the mind uses immediately in the performance of the actions termed animal; but it seems not improbable that *the sensorium commune, properly so called, extends to the medulla oblongata, the crura cerebri and cerebelli, even to part of the thalami optici, and to the whole spinal marrow, in a word, as widely as the origin of the nerves.* That the sensorium commune extends to the spinal marrow, we learn from the motions remaining in decapitated animals, which could not take place without the consent and co-operation of the nerves arising from the spinal marrow; for if a decapitated frog be pricked, not only does it retract the punctured part, but it crawls

retrahit, verum etiam repit, et saltat, quod absque consensu nervorum sensoriorum et motoriorum fieri nequit, cujus consensus sedes in medulla spinali, superstite sensorii communis parte, sit oportet.

Impressionum sensoriarum in motorias reflexio, quæ in sensorio communi fit, non peragitur juxta solas leges physicas, ubi angulus reflexionis æqualis est angulo incidentiæ, et ubi, quanta fit actio, tanta etiam sequitur reactio; sed leges peculiares, a natura in pulpam medullarem sensorii quasi scriptas, sequitur ista reflexio quas ex solis effectibus tantam noscere, neutiquam vero assequi ingenio nostro valemus. GENERALIS TAMEN LEX, QUA COMMUNE SENSORIUM IMPRESSIONES SENSORIAS IN MOTORIAS REFLECTIT, EST NOSTRI CONSERVATIO: ITA UT IMPRESSIONES EXTERNAS CORPORI NOSTRO NOCITURAS SEQUANTUR CERTÆ IMPRESSIONES MOTORIÆ, MOTUS PRODUCTURAE EO COLLIMANTES, UT NOCUMENTUM A CORPORE NOSTRO ARCEATUR, AMOVEATURQUE; ET VICE

---

and leaps, which could not be without the consent of the sensorial and motor nerves, of which consent the seat must be in the spinal marrow, the part of the sensorium commune remaining.

The reflection of sensorial into motory impressions, which takes place in the sensorium commune, does not obey mere physical laws, where the angle of reflexion is equal to the angle of incidence, and where action and reaction are equal, but it follows peculiar laws written, as it were, by nature, in the medullary pulp of the sensorium, which we can know only by their effects, and not discover by our imagination. Nevertheless, A GENERAL LAW, ACCORDING TO WHICH THE SENSORIUM COMMUNE REFLECTS SENSORIAL INTO MOTOR IMPRESSIONS, IS OUR PRESERVATION: SO THAT CERTAIN MOTORY IMPRESSIONS FOLLOW EXTERNAL IMPRESSIONS HURTFUL TO THE BODY, PRODUCING MOTIONS TENDING TO

VERSA IMPRESSIONES EXTERNAS SEU SENSORIAS, NOBIS PROFUTURAS, SEQUANTUR IMPRESSIONES INTERNÆ SEU MOTORIÆ, MOTUS PRODUCTURÆ EO TENDENTES, UT GRATUS ILLE STATUS ULTRO CONSERVETUR. Hanc generalem reflexionum sensorii communis legem probant certe plurima exempla, quæ adduci possent, quorum pauca tantum adduxisse sufficiet. Irritatio in membrana narium interna facta excitat sternutationem, quia impressio illa ab irritatione in nervis olfactoriis facta per eos ad sensorium commune defertur, ibi certa lege reflectitur in nervos motorios, musculis respirationi dicatis prospicientes, et per hos validam expirationem per nares producit, qua per aërem vi transeuntem irritamentum avellitur, et ejicitur. Ita fit, ubi irritatio in aspera arteria per micam cibi, vel guttulam potus illapsam causatur: facit hæc irritatio ad sensorium commune delata, et ibidem in nervos respirationis motui dicatos reflexa,

---

WARD OFF AND REMOVE THE SOURCE OF INJURY; AND, ON THE CONTRARY, INTERNAL OR MOTOR IMPRESSIONS FOLLOW EXTERNAL OR SENSORIAL IMPRESSIONS BENEFICIAL TO US, PRODUCING MOTIONS CALCULATED TO PERPETUATE THAT BENEFIT. Many examples certainly prove this general law of the reflections of the sensorium commune, of which it will be sufficient to adduce a few. Irritation of the internal membrane of the nostrils excites sneezing, because that impression, made by irritation of the olfactory nerves, is by them carried to the sensorium commune, is there reflected, according to a certain law, upon motor nerves going to the muscles appropriated to respiration, and, through these, produces a forcible expiration through the nose, in which, by the air forcibly passing, the irritation is removed. So it happens when any irritation is caused to the wind-pipe by a crumb of bread or a drop of liquid falling into it: this irritation, carried to the sensorium commune, and thence reflected upon the nerves appropriated to

ut excitetur valida tussis, aptissimum ad expellendum irritamentum remedium, quæ prius non desinit, donec irritamentum ejectum non fuerit. Si amicus digito suo appropinquat ad oculum nostrum, licet persuasissimus nihil mali nobis inferendum esse, tamen jam impressio illa per opticum nervum ad sensorium commune delata, in sensorio ita reflectitur in nervos palpebrarum motui dicatos, ut *nollentibus* claudantur palpebræ, et arceant molestum digiti ad occulum attactum. Hæc et innumera, quæ afferi possent, exempla manifeste ostendunt, quantopere reflexio sensoriarum impressionum in motorias per sensorium commune facienda conservationem nostri corporis respiciat. Propterea recte etiam Illustr. Tissotus actionem sensorii communis illis viribus adnumerat, quarum summa atque connubium naturam corporis nostri viventis constituit.

Cum itaque *præcipua functio sensorii communis*

---

respiratory motion, excites a forcible cough, the most apt remedy for expelling the irritant, which does not cease until that irritant is removed. If a friend approaches our eye with his finger, although we are persuaded that no harm will be done to us, yet that impression carried by the optic nerve to the sensorium commune, is in the sensorium so reflected upon the nerves appropriated to the motion of the eyelids, that the palpebræ are *involuntarily* closed so as to avoid the contact of the finger. These and innumerable other examples that might be adduced, show manifestly how much the reflection of sensorial into motor impressions by the sensorium commune regards the preservation of our body. On this account, Tissot properly enumerates the action of the sensorium commune amongst those powers of which the end and union constitute the nature of our living body.

As, therefore, *the principal function of the sensorium commune*

consistat in reflexione impressionum sensoriarum in motorias, notandum est, quod ISTA REFLEXIO VEL ANIMA INSCIA, VEL VERO ANIMA CONSCIA FIAT. Motus cordis, ventriculi, et intestinorum certe ab animæ conscientia nequaquam pendent, cum tamen nullus motus muscularis cieri possit, nisi stimulus nervis sensoriis applicatus in nervos motorios reflexione quadam transeat, et musculi contractionem cieat, tunc certum est reflexionem impressionum istis motibus excitandis aptarum, si in sensorio communi fiunt, fieri sine animæ conscientia. Verum quæritur, utrum istæ impressiones ad sensorium commune usque adscendant reflectendæ, an vero sine hac ambage citius in gangliis, unde plurimos nervos istæ partes habent, reflectantur? Hac de re postea adhuc agetur. Sed fieri tamen reflexiones impressionum sensoriarum in motorias in ipso sensorio communi anima prorsus nescia docent actiones quædam

---

consists in the reflection of sensorial into motor impressions, it is to be observed, that THIS REFLECTION TAKES PLACE WHETHER THE MIND BE CONSCIOUS OR UNCONSCIOUS OF IT. The motion of the heart, of the stomach, and of the intestines, certainly in no respect depend on the consciousness of the mind; but as no muscular motion can be excited, unless a stimulus applied to the sensorial nerves passes by a certain reflection to the motor nerves, and excites muscular contraction, so it is certain that the reflection of impressions proper for inducing these motions, if they take place in the sensorium commune, takes place without the consciousness of the mind. But it is asked whether these impressions ascend to the sensorium commune, to be reflected, or whether, without making this circuit, they are more quickly reflected by the ganglia, whence these parts have many nerves. More on this point hereafter. But that the reflections of sensorial into motor impressions take place

in apoplecticis, quibus tota conscientia ablata est, superstites: nam et pulsu forti gaudent, et valide respirant, et etiam manum elevant, locoque affecto persæpe admovent inscii. Agit etiam sensorium commune sine animæ conscientia convulsivos motus epilepticorum producendo, et etiam illas, quæ in profundo somno sepultis præter motum cordis et respirium aliquando observantur, artuum punctorum et leviter vellicatorum retractiones. Huc quoque spectant omnes motus, qui in corpore decapitati hominis aut alius animalis aliquo tempore supersunt, et vellicato corpore, præprimis vero medulla spinali, excitantur, qui certe sine conscientia animæ fiunt, et per residuam sensorii communis partem, quæ in medulla spinali est, reguntur. OMNES ISTÆ ACTIONES EX ORGANISMO ET PHYSICIS LEGIBUS, SENSORIO COMMUNI PROPRIIS, FLUUNT, SUNTQUE PROPTEREA SPON-

---

quite unconsciously in the sensorium commune, we learn from certain actions remaining in apoplectic patients, in whom all consciousness is destroyed; for they have a strong pulse, breathe strongly, and often even raise the hand unconsciously to the part affected. The sensorium commune acts also without consciousness in producing the convulsive motions of epileptic patients, and even those retractions of the limbs when slightly pricked or pinched, which are sometimes observed in profound sleep, besides motion of the heart and respiration. To these we must add all those motions which for some time remain in the body of a decapitated man, or other animal, and are excited by pinching the body, but especially the spinal marrow, which certainly occur without consciousness, and are governed by the residual part of the sensorium commune, which is in the spinal marrow. ALL THESE ACTIONS ARISE FROM THE ORGANISATION AND PHYSICAL LAWS PROPER TO THE SENSORIUM COMMUNE, AND ARE, THEREFORE, SPONTANEOUS AND AUTO-

TANEÆ AC AUTOMATICÆ. Illæ actiones, quæ in corpore animali fiunt anima conscia, vel sunt tales, in quas anima voluntatis suæ nullum habet imperium, vel vero tales, quas anima coercere et impedire pro libitu potest: illæ cum solo sensorio communi, quatenus ab anima non dependet, regantur, etiam nihilominus, quam quæ inscia mente fiunt, automaticæ actiones sunt; talis est sternutatio a stimulo naribus applicito, tussis a stimulo traheæ illapso, vomitus a titillatione faucium aut emetico assumto, tremores ac convulsiones in chorea S. Viti, et in paroxismo febris intermittentis, etc. Actiones vero, quas anima suo imperio dirigit ac moderatur, quamvis etiam in iisdem producendis sensorium commune suam partem habeat, vocamus nihilominus animales, non automaticas.

MATIC. Those actions, which take place in the animal body with consciousness, are either such, that the mind has no power over its will, or such as the mind can coerce or impede at will: the former, as they are ruled by the sensorium commune alone, in as far as it does not depend upon the mind, are also automatic actions, not less than those which are performed unconsciously; such are sneezing from a stimulus applied to the nostrils, cough from a stimulus applied to the trachea, vomiting from irritation of the fauces, or from an emetic, tremor and convulsions in chorea S. Viti, and in the paroxysms of intermittent fever, &c. But the actions which the mind directs and moderates by its power, although the sensorium commune has its part in producing them, we call, nevertheless, animal, not automatic.

NOTE RESPECTING THE OPINIONS OF MR. MAYO, SIR G. BLANE, AND M. LEGALLOIS.

MR. MAYO, in his Anatomical Commentaries, published in 1823, implicitly followed the opinions of Whytt and Prochaska—imputing to the organization, in the production of these phenomena, sensation and involition.

In No. II. of that work, page 17, he says, "It is clear that *an influence, independent of the will*, occasionally throws voluntary muscles into action, as appears in tetanus, and other spasmodic disorders; and is shown remarkably in the physiological experiment of irritating the skin on the lower extremities, after the division of the spinal cord in the back, when the occurrence of action limited to the muscles of the lower extremities evinces that *a connexion* exists, *independently of the will*, between SENTIENT SURFACES and the action of voluntary MUSCLES. I have varied this experiment by dividing the spinal cord at once in the neck and in the back, upon which three unconnected nervous centres exist; and the division of the skin in either part (and especially at the soles of the feet in the two hinder portions) produces a convulsive action of the muscles in that part. The same influence may then possibly regulate the unconscious actions to which these remarks relate."

In page 138 of the same Part, he says, "*An influence* may be propagated from the SENTIENT NERVES of a part to their correspondent NERVES OF MOTION, through the intervention of that part alone of the nervous centre, to which they are mutually attached. Thus in vertebral animals, in which alone the fact is questionable, when the spinal cord has been divided in two places, an injury of the skin of either region is followed by a distinct muscular action in that part. Again: if the brain is quickly removed from the head of a pigeon, leaving only the crura cerebri, together with the tubercles and the second and third nerve, on pinching the second nerve, the iris contracts."

In the last edition (1837) of his "Outlines of Physiology," he says, "Each segment of the double cord, from which a pair of nerves arises, has in itself a mechanism of SENSATION and INSTINCTIVE ACTION, comparable to the parallel parts in articulate animals. The proof of this is contained in the following remarkable experiments made upon the body, a few seconds after it has been deprived of life. If the spinal cord be then divided in the middle of the neck, and again in the middle of the back, upon irritating a SENTIENT ORGAN connected with either isolated segment, muscular action is produced; if the sole of the foot is pricked, the foot is suddenly retracted, with the same gesture as it would have been during life; that is to say, a SENTIENT ORGAN is excited, and an irritation is propagated through the

SENTIENT NERVE, to the isolated segment of spinal marrow, when it gives rise to some change, which is followed by an impulse along the VOLUNTARY NERVES (!) to the muscles of the part."

Mr. Mayo, having, in all the statements now quoted, spoken only of "sensation," "sentient organs," "sentient surfaces," "sentient nerves," and of "instinctive action," "independence of the will," &c. the expression "*voluntary nerves*," here used is an inconsistency and probably an oversight. The following, however, is quite inexplicable on any supposition. "The same view and the same facts, *carefully distinguished from the agency of sensation and volition*, have been put forward in the former editions (as in the present) of my Outlines of Physiology."*

With the motions which continue in decapitated animals, particularly under irritation applied to the surface, SIR G. BLANE connected the phenomena of instinctive actions, as the first acts of inspiration and of sucking, and *inferred that such* INSTINCTIVE OR AUTOMATIC MOVEMENTS, *being independent on the brain, are* NOT DEPENDENT ON SENSATION.

In the phenomena previously described, M. LEGALLOIS *asserted the existence both of* SENSATION *and of*

* Page 334 of that work.

VOLUNTARY MOTION*—being the very reverse of the doctrine of Dr. Marshall Hall, documents relative to which are now to follow.

* Si, au lieu de détruire la moëlle on y fait des sections transversales, les parties correspondantes à chaque segment de la moëlle jouissent du SENTIMENT et du MOUVEMENT VOLONTAIRE, mais sans aucune harmonie et d'une manière aussi indépendante entre elles que si on eût coupeé transversalement tout le corps de l'animal aux mêmes endroits; en un mot il y a dans ce cas autant de centres de sensations, bien distincts, qu'on a fait de segmens à la moëlle.—Works, T. I, p. 135.

THESE MOTIONS INDEPENDENT OF SENSATION AND VOLITION.

BY MARSHALL HALL, M.D. F.R.S.

Date of Publication—1832.

First communication made to the Zoological Society, November the 27th, 1832.—*The following is an extract from the Proceedings of the Committee of Science:*

A PAPER was read, containing 'a brief account of a particular function of the nervous system,' in which Dr. Marshall Hall detailed a series of experiments tending to prove the existence of *a source of muscular action distinct from all those hitherto noticed by physiologists, viz. volition, the irritation of the motor nerves in some part of their origin or course, or that of the muscles themselves.* The peculiarity of this motion he stated to consist in its being excited by irritation of the extreme portion of the sentient nerves, whence the impression is conveyed through the corresponding portion of brain and spinal marrow as a centre, to the extremities of the motor nerves.

The animals experimented on were salamanders, frogs and turtles. In the first of these, the tail, entirely separated from the body, moved as in the living animal, on being excited by the point of a needle passed lightly over its surface. The motion ceased on destroying the spinal marrow within the caudal *vertebræ.* The head of a frog having been removed, and the spine divided between the third and fourth *vertebræ,* an eye of the separated head was touched: it was retracted and the eye-lid closed,—a similar movement being observed in the other eye. On removing the brain, these phenomena ceased. On pinching the skin, or the toe of one of the anterior extremities, the whole of this portion of the animal moved. On destroying the spinal marrow, this phenomenon also ceased. Precisely similar effects were observed on pinching the skin or toe of one of the posterior extremities; and on removing the last portion of the spinal marrow, this phenomenon ceased. The head of the turtle continues to move long after its separation from the body: on pinching the eye-lid, it is forcibly closed, the mouth is opened, and the membrane expanded under the lower jaw descends as in respiration. On pinching any part of the skin of the body, extremities, or tail, the animal moves. The posterior extremities and tail being separated together, the former were immovable; the latter moved on the application of the flame of a lighted taper to the skin. Those extremities had no connection with the spinal marrow. All movement ceased in the tail also, on withdrawing the spinal marrow from its canal.

'Three things,' Dr. Hall observes, 'are plain from these observations: 1. That the nerves of sensibility are impressible in portions of an animal separated from the rest; in the head, in the upper part of the trunk, in the lower part of the trunk: 2. that motions similar to voluntary motions follow these impressions made upon the sentient nerves: and 3. that the presence of the spinal marrow is essential as the central and cementing link between the sentient and motor nerves.'

Dr. Hall then proceeded to adduce another series of experiments still more conclusive. If a frog be made to swallow a watery solution of opium, it becomes affected with symptoms very similar to those of tetanus and hydrophobia; the body and limbs become rigidly extended; but besides this state of spasm, the cutaneous nerves become extremely susceptive, and the motor nerves extremely excitative; a shake, a touch, a breath of air even, induces spasmodic movements of the body and limbs. A frog made tetanic by opium was decapitated and divided just below the third *vertebra.* The eyes continued drawn in, and no motion could be detected on irritating the eye, eye-lid, or skin. But both the anterior and posterior parts remained tetanic as before. The limbs were moved in the same spasmodic manner by the same slight impressions. The exalted condition of the function of the sentient and motor nerves continued in each part. All was changed, on removing the brain and the respective portions of spinal marrow. The eyes were immovable, but no longer retracted; the muscles of the limbs were flaccid, and there was no evidence of irritability in the sentient nerves.

'These experiments,' Dr. Hall continued, 'appear to me to establish a property or function of the nervous system,—of the sentient and motor nerves,—distinct from sensation and voluntary or instinctive motion. However doubtful this conclusion might appear in reference to the first series of experiments upon the animal in its natural state, it can scarcely admit of doubt when we compare with them the phenomena observed in the frog made tetanic by opium. In this case, the contraction of the muscles is plainly *not* the result of volition; and it obeys the same laws, in regard to its continuance and extinction, as the similar function or property in its natural and unexalted state. Neither does it arise from the irritation of the motor nerves, or muscular fibre; for it ceases on removing the spinal marrow, while the property of irritability continues unimpaired after the destruction of the nervous centre. I conclude, then, that *there is a property of the sentient and motory system of nerves which is independent of sensation and volition;—a property of the motor nerves independent of immoderate irritation;—a property which attaches itself to any part of an animal, the corresponding portion of the brain and spinal marrow of which is entire.* This property is capable of exaltation, in the frog, from the influence of opium, and doubtless of strychnine; and I may add, that it is diminished or extinguished by the hydrocyanic acid. It is naturally greatest in animals of lowest *sensibility*, as the cold-blooded.'

With regard to the office performed by this property of the nervous system in the animal economy, Dr. Hall stated that it appeared especially to preside over all those functions which, from appearing neither exclusively voluntary nor independent of the will, have been designated mixed. That the function of respiration is of this kind, he considered plain, from the phenomena presented by the separated head of the turtle, in which the submaxillary integuments became alternately inflated and contracted as in ordinary respiration. The actions of coughing, sneezing, vomiting, &c., are of the same kind. So, apparently, is the singular effect produced by tickling. Of all the parts of the human frame, the *larynx* and the *anus* appear to be most under the influence of this peculiar power. No part is so impatient of irritation as the former; none so much in need of automatic action as the latter, with the other sphincters. These very parts are subject, moreover, to peculiar morbid affections of this function: in regard to the larynx, it is observed in some affections of dangerous tendency referred to spasm: in the sphincters it is seen in those singular and painful affections termed strangury and tenesmus. There are also peculiar affections of the system of voluntary muscles referrible to the same property. In hydrophobia and tetanus, in each of which the extremities of the sentient nerves have been wounded, there is a peculiar exaltation of this function: the morbid action appears to be propagated to the spinal marrow; and then along the motor nerves, producing those dreadful sensations and spasms so fearfully characteristic of these affections. The least external shock or impression is terrible; the immediate muscular contractions are intolerable.

THESE MOTIONS REFLEX OR EXCITO-MOTORY.

BY MARSHALL HALL, M.D. F.R.S.

Date of Publication—1834.

Second Communication made to the Zoological Society, and read on August the 12*th,* 1834.—*The following Account is extracted from the "Proceedings."*

DR. MARSHALL HALL showed some experiments in the decapitated TURTLE. Irritation of the nostrils, *larynx* and spinal marrow, induced acts of inspiration; that of the fins and tail induced movements of the other parts respectively.

But the principal object of Dr. Hall was to show that irritation of the nerves themselves equally induced movements of the limbs, &c. **WHEN EITHER THE SENTIENT OR THE MOTORY BRANCH OF THE LATERAL SPINAL NERVES WAS STIMULATED, MOTIONS WERE INDUCED IN ALL THE LIMBS.** Dr. Hall stated that a movement of inspiration and deglutition was caused in the *donkey* by irritation of the eighth pair of nerves. It has been already stated that irritation of the nostrils, or the branches of the fifth pair of nerves, induced inspiratory acts in the *turtle*. From these and other facts, Dr. Hall is induced to consider the functions of these two nerves as similar. He further observed that both are nerves of secretion, and that both are muscular nerves—if the minor portion of the fifth, and the accessory, be included—as well as *excitors of respiration*; the fifth differs chiefly in being sentient, being distributed to external as well as internal surfaces. With the fifth and eighth, Dr. Hall associates other spinal nerves. He considers *respiration as a part of a general function of the nervous system, which presides over the larynx, the pharynx, sphincters, ejaculators, &c., to which he has given the name of reflex, from its consisting of impressions carried to and from the medulla oblongata and medulla spinalis.* Some illustrations of this function were given by Dr. Hall at the Meeting of the Committee of Science and Correspondence, on November 27, 1832 (Proceedings, Part II, p. 190), and further illustrations of it have formed the subject of a paper by him, which has since been published in the 'Philosophical Transactions.' *The experiments shown on the present occasion demonstrate the existence of a series of physiological facts at variance with the law laid down by M. Müller*, in his paper entitled 'Nouvelles Expériences sur l'Effet que produit l'Irritation Mécanique et Galvanique sur les Racines des Nerfs Spinaux: par Jean Müller, Professeur à l'Université de Bonn,' and published in the 'Annales des Sciences Naturelles,' tom. xxiii. (1831), p. 95, viz.: "Il suit encore qu'il y a des nerfs qui n'ont point de force *motrice* ou *tonique*, qui ne peuvent jamais occasionner des mouvemens par eux-mêmes, qu'ils soient irrités par l'action galvanique ou mécanique, et qui ne conduisent le courant galvanique que passivement, comme toutes les parties molles humides; qu'il y a en revanche des *nerfs moteurs* ou *toniques* (*nervi motorii* seu *tonici*) qui montrent à chaque indication médiate ou immédiate leur *force tonique, qui agit toujours dans la direction des branches des nerfs et qui n'agit jamais en arrière.*' *In Dr. Hall's experiments,* THE INFLUENCE FIRST PURSUED AN 'ARRIÈRE' COURSE TO THE SPINAL MARROW, *being afterwards reflected upon the muscles.*

Dr. Hall next observed, in regard to respiration, that, whilst Sir Charles Bell contends that it is involuntary, and Mr. Mayo that it is voluntary, the old doctrine of its being mixed, or partaking of both properties, is the true one. He founded this view upon the following facts:

1. If the *cerebrum* be removed, respiration continues as an involuntary function through the agency of the eighth pair of nerves.

2. If the eighth pair be divided, respiration equally continues, but as an act of volition; but

3. If the *cerebrum* be first removed, and the eighth pair be then divided, respiration ceases on the instant. Volition is first removed with the *cerebrum;* the influence of the eighth pair is then removed by its division. The two sources of the mixed or double function being both cut off, the function ceases.

Dr. Hall explains and reconciles in this manner the difficult and apparently contradictory facts,—that the *medulla oblongata* alone, above the origin of the eighth pair of nerves, or the eighth pair of nerves themselves, may be divided, without arresting the respiration; but that the medulla oblongata cannot be divided at the origin of these nerves without arresting the respiration instantly. In the first case, the agency of volition is alone removed, and the respiration continues through the influence of the eighth pair; in the second, that of the eighth pair is removed, and the respiration continues as a function of volition; but in the third, both influences are destroyed at once, and with them the mixed or double function.

The same mixed or double character belongs to the other parts of the reflex function, as that of the *larynx*, the sphincters, the ejaculators. All the organs of the reflex function are also alike impressed through the medium of the mental affections or passions.

The course of the influence which constitutes the reflex function must be divided into the incident, or that into the medulla, and the reflected, or that from the medulla. The nerves which conduct the incident impression have, hitherto, received no designation; the others constitute a part of the system of muscular nerves. To the former class belong nerves which doubtless supply the *larynx* with its impressibility by carbonic acid, &c. &c., and hitherto undescribed, untraced; to the latter, the superior and inferior laryngeals: to the former belong the fifth, in the nostrils, in the face,—the eighth in the lungs, &c.; to the latter the respiratory nerves: to the former, nerves hitherto undescribed of the sphincters, ejaculators, &c.; to the latter, the muscular nerves supplying these parts.

SYNOPTICAL VIEW OF THE EXCITO-MOTORY SYSTEM.

BY MARSHALL HALL, M.D. F.R.S.

Date of Publication—1839.

TABLE I.

Anatomy of the True Spinal System.

I. *The Incident Motor Branches.*

1. *The Trifacial, arising from—*
   1. *The Eye-lashes.*
   2. *The Alæ Nasi.*
   3. *The Nostril.*
   4. *The Fauces.*
   5. *The Face.*
2. *The Pneumogastric, from*
   1. *The Pharynx.*
   2. *The Larynx.*
   3. *The Bronchia.*
   4. *The Cardia,—Kidney, and Liver.*
3. *The Posterior Spinal, arising from*
   1. *The General Surface.*
   2. *The Glans Penis vel Clitoridis.*
   3. *The Anus.*
   4. *The Cervix Vesicæ.*
   5. *The Cervix Uteri.*

II. *The True Medulla Oblongata and Medulla Spinalis, the Centre of the System.*

III. *The Reflex, Motor Branches*

1. *The Trochlearis* } *Oculi.*
2. *The Abducens* } *Oculi.*
3. *The Minor portion of the Fifth*
4. *The Facial, distributed to*
   1. *The Orbicularis.*
   2. *The Levator Alæ Nasi.*
5. *The Pneumogastric or its Accessory.*
   1. *The Pharyngeal.*
   2. *The Œsophageal and Cardiac*
   3. *The Laryngeal.*
   4. *The Bronchial, &c.*
6. *The Myo-glossal.*
7. *The Spinal, distributed to*
   1. *The Diaphragm, and to*
   2. *The Intercostal &* } *Muscles.*
   3. *The Abdominal* } *Muscles.*
8. *The Sacral, distributed to*
   1. *The Sphincters.*
   2. *The Expulsors, the Ejaculators, the Fallopian Tubes, the Uterus, &c.*

TABLE II.

Physiology of the True Spinal System.

I. *The Excited Action—*

1. *Of the Eyes, the Eye-lids; and of the Iris?*
2. *Of the Orifices.* { 1. *The Larynx.* 2. *The Pharynx.* }
3. *Of the Ingestion.*
    1. *Of the Food.*
        1. *In Suction;*
        2. *In Deglutition.*
    2. *Of the Air, or Respiration.*
    3. *Of the Semen, or Conception.*
4. *Of Exclusion.*
5. *Of the Expulsors, or of Egestion.*
    1. *Of the Fæces;*
    2. *Of the Urine;*
    3. *Of the Perspiration;*
    4. *Of the Semen;*
    5. *Of the Fœtus.*
6. *Of the Sphincters.*

II. *The Direct Action or Influence—*

I. *In the Tone.* } *of the Muscular System.*
II. *In the Irritability.* }

TABLE III.

Pathology of the True Spinal System.

I. *Diseases of the Incident Nerves.*

I. 1. *Dental* 2. *Gastric* 3. *Intestinal*	*Irritation in Infants.*	1. *The Crowing Inspiration.* 2. *Strabismus, Spasm of the Fingers and Toes; Strangury; Tenesmus; &c.* 3. *Convulsion.* 4. *Paralysis?*
II. 1. *Gastric* 2. *Intestinal* 3. *Uterine*	*Irritation in Adults.*	I. *Hysteria.* II. *Asthma.* III. *Vomiting; Hiccup; &c.* IV. *Epilepsy.* V. *Puerperal Convulsion; &c.*

III. *Traumatic Tetanus.*

IV. *Hydrophobia, &c.*

II. *Diseases of the Spinal Marrow itself.*

I. *Inflammation and other Diseases.*

II. *Diseases of the Vertebræ.*

III. *Counter-pressure, &c. in Diseases within the Cranium.*

IV. *Centric Epilepsy.*

V. *Centric Tetanus.*

VI. *Convulsions from Loss of Blood; &c.*

III. *Diseases of the Reflex or Motor Nerves.*

I. *Spasm.*

1. *Spasmodic Tic.*
2. *Torticollis.*
3. *Contracted Limbs; &c.*

II. *Paralysis.*

COINCIDENCE OF DR. HALL'S AND PROFESSOR MULLER'S OBSERVATIONS.

In his Manual of Physiology, Book III. Chapter III. Müller makes the following statement:—

Die hier zu untersuchenden Phänomene sind fast zu gleicher Zeit von mir und Marshall Hall beobachtet worden. Wie der grösste Theil der Nervenphysik, wie sie hier gegeben wird, bereits seit mehreren Jahren vollendet war, so war auch dieses Capitel über die reflectirten Bewegungen nach Empfindungen seit mehreren Jahren schon fast gerade so niedergeschrieben, wie es hier gegeben wird. Dass diese Erklärung aufrichtig ist, geht aus der ersten Abtheilung dieses Handbuchs hervor, welches im Früchling 1833 erschien, und welches p. 333—335, schon die Grundsätze über die reflectirten Bewegungen und Empfindungen aus Beobachtungen

---

The phenomena here investigated were observed by me and Marshall Hall almost at the same time. As the greater part of the physiology of the nerves, here delivered, was concluded many years ago, so was this subject of the reflected motions after sensation, and that almost as plainly as here stated. That this explanation is perfectly ingenuous, is evident from the first part of this manual, which appeared in the spring of 1833, and which, p. 333—335, explained from observation the principles of the reflex motions

entwickelt, welche hier weiter ausgeführt werden. Merkwürdiger Weise sind dieselben Ideen selbst mit denselben Beispielen und Beobachtungen an narcotisirten Thieren in demselben Jahre von Marshall Hall in den Philos. Transact. 1833, vorgetragen worden. Obgleich diese Ideen unabhängig von einander entstanden waren, so ist doch die grosse Uebereinstimmung in den Beobachtungen und Erklärungen nicht schwer zu begreifen, wenn man bedenkt, wie die Ausbildung der Nervenphysik eine Consequenz erlangt hat, welche die entferntesten Beobachter gleichzeitig zu gleichen neuen Beobachtungen und Erklärungen führen kann.

In a note, however, on the English translation, page 707, Müller says:—

"The paper of Dr. Hall, which is here referred to, appeared in the second part of the Philosophical Transactions for 1833. I first stated my views in the first edition of the first part of this work, which appeared in the spring of that year, in the chapter on the respiratory movements, and more fully in the second part of the work in the following year, 1834,

---

and sensations, which are here further developed. In a remarkable manner, the same ideas, with the same examples and observations on narcotized animals, were advanced by Marshall Hall in the same year, in the Philos. Transact. 1833. Though these ideas occurred to us independently of each other, still the great agreement between our observations and explanations is not difficult to be understood, when we reflect how the cultivation of the physiology of the nerves has attained a sequence, which may lead the most remote observers at the same time to similar new observations and explanations.

after Dr. Hall's paper had appeared. *A paper by Dr. Hall had, however, been read at the Zoological Society on this subject, in* 1832: HE HAS, THEREFORE, THE PRIORITY."

In a Postscript to his Memoirs on the Nervous System, 1837, Dr. Hall says:—"During the *four years,* which elapsed between the publication of my first and second Memoirs, the subject of this volume was treated with opposition or neglect. That it has been rescued from this treatment is, I believe, mainly due to the just influence of an illustrious foreigner. The sanction of Professor Müller to the truth, importance, and originality of this discovery, I feel to be of the utmost value to the progress of the Inquiry.

"Prof. Müller includes the *brain,* and even the *sympathetic* with the spinal marrow, as agents of the *reflex motions;* and he does *not* distinguish the *principle* of these motions from *sensation.* It is almost needless to repeat, that I have, on the contrary, demonstrated that the *spinal marrow,* distinguished from the *brain,* from the spinal *chord,* and from the *sympathetic,* is the sole organic seat of this function; that the principle of this function is, at oncc, *distinct* from sensation, and *identical* with another property of the nervous system,—long imperfectly known to physiologists, yet hitherto, strange to say, *unapplied* to Physiology,—designated by Haller, the *vis nervosa,* and by Prof. Müller himself, the *vis motoria,* and now the excito-motory property or power.

"I have discovered and demonstrated new modes of action of this power,—modes at variance with the views of Haller, and the *laws* laid down by Prof. Müller, and have *identified* it with the principle which acts when, the spinal marrow being divided, one of the lower extremities is stimulated,—a second principle known to physiologists, yet *unapplied* to physiology! I have made it probable that it acts through *a true spinal marrow,* and *a distinct and peculiar system of nerves,* the existence of which had not been even suspected before.

"I have designated the system by terms which Prof. Müller, entertaining the opinions which he does, could not use. The terms *true spinal* and *excito-motory,* express views at variance with those held by Prof. Müller.

"Lastly, I have traced the excito-motory principle through its anatomical, physiological, pathological, and therapeutic relations, in a manner and degree not attempted by Prof. Müller."

SUPPOSED INTERFERENCE OF DR. HALL'S AND PROCHASKA'S OPINIONS.

On this subject, scarcely one sentence is necessary. Sensation is the basis of Prochaska's doctrine; it is utterly rejected by Hall: Prochaska extends his sensorium commune to the encephalon; Hall entirely excludes that as well as the cerebral nerves, and limits it to a distinct and true spinal marrow, the sole centre of a system of incident, excitor, and reflex motor nerves—the exclusive seat of the excito-motory power, on which alone depend the ingestors, the expulsors, the orifices, the sphincters. Argument on this subject would be absurd.

THESE MOTIONS SOMETIMES SENSITIVE AND ALWAYS INVOLUNTARY; PARTIAL RETURN TO THE DOCTRINE OF WHYTT.*

BY J. MULLER, M.D.

Date of Publication—1833.

[FROM the "Manual of Physiology" it would be useless to make any long extract, seeing that it is in the hands of every student, or ought to be so, even if he had no other book on the subject. No more, therefore, is here quoted from it than is necessary to express the general character of its doctrine on this subject as given by the author himself, and to permit a very brief comparison of it with those which have preceded.]

WHEN IMPRESSIONS MADE BY THE ACTION OF EXTERNAL STIMULI ON SENSITIVE NERVES GIVE RISE TO MOTIONS IN OTHER PARTS, THESE ARE NEVER THE RESULT OF THE DIRECT RE-ACTION OF THE SENSITIVE AND MOTOR FIBRES OF THE NERVES ON EACH OTHER; THE IRRITATION IS CONVEYED BY THE SENSITIVE FIBRES TO THE BRAIN AND SPINAL CORD, AND IS BY THESE COMMUNICATED TO THE MOTOR FIBRES.

The view which I take of the matter is the follow-

* The precise extent to which this takes place appears from the 1st paragraph here printed in small capitals. It indeed scarcely differs from the last paragraph quoted from Whytt in page 121.

ing:—irritation of *sensitive fibres* of a spinal nerve excites primarily a *centripetal action* of the nervous principle, conveying the impression to the spinal cord; *if the centripetal action can then be continued to the sensorium commune, a true sensation is the result; if, on account of division of the spinal cord, it cannot be communicated to the sensorium, it still exerts its whole influence upon the spinal cord; in both cases, a reflex motor action may be the result.* In the first case, the centripetal action excites, at the same time, SENSATION; in the latter case, it does not, but is still adequate to the production of REFLEX MOTION, or centrifugal reflection.

Dr. Hall's theory differs from that of Whytt, as well as from my own, and is peculiar. In the first place, he limits the phenomenon of reflex action to the spinal nerves, and denies to the cerebral nerves of special sense the power of exciting them. He supposes the reflex motor actions to be in no case excited by sensation, nor even by means of the sensitive nervous fibres. He maintains the existence of special nerves, or nervous fibres, endowed with the "excito-motory" function; and the reflex action he supposes to be conveyed, not by the nerves of spontaneous motion, but by special fibres, which he calls "reflecto-motory."—The posterior roots of the spinal nerves, and nerves of the medulla oblongata, Dr. Hall teaches, contain sensitive and excito-motory fibres; the anterior roots, spontano-motory and reflecto-motory fibres.

DOCUMENTS RELATIVE TO THE GANGLIA, ETC.

ABSTRACT OF

GENERAL PROPOSITIONS ON THE FUNCTIONS OF THE GANGLIONIC SYSTEM.

BY JAMES COPLAND, M.D.

Read at the Medical Society of London—in 1820.

*It was subsequently printed in Appendix to the Author's Translation of Richerand's Elements of Physiology.**

It may be proper to remark, that these inferences were deduced from numerous dissections of individual subjects belonging to the different classes of animals, and from several experiments made in order to ascertain the extent of function which this system of nerves performs.

In all the more perfect animals, the ganglia and their various distributions, as far as they can be traced by the senses, even when aided by powerful glasses and minute dissection, are entirely different from the nerves derived from the brain and spinal chord, in their texture, colour, consistence, mode of ramification and distribution; and they supply very

* It is inserted here, as being, up to the period of its publication, the most comprehensive and original view of the ganglionic system.

different organs and textures from those to which the cerebral and spinal nerves are distributed.

Not only in the lowest order of animals may the ganglial nerves be traced before the voluntary or sentient class of nerves come into existence, but also in the embryos of the higher animals the ganglia may be distinguished before any traces of a spinal marrow or of a brain can be perceived.*

The ganglial nerves cannot be supposed to originate in either the brain or spinal marrow:—1st, because they are observed in the lowest animals, which possess neither brain nor spinal chord; 2dly, because they may be distinguished in embryos before either one or the other nervous mass can be traced; and 3dly, because they are never wanting in the fœtal state,—whereas not only have the brain and spinal marrow been individually wanting, but the same fœtus has been found entirely without both.

The difference between this class of nerves and those of animal life, is not evinced only by their respective appearances, by the general distribution of the former throughout the animal creation, by the history of the embryal fœtus, and by the phenomena exhibited by monsters; but it is also apparent from the very different effects which are observed in them, as respects both the living and dead subject, on the application of various excitants and re-agents.†

* Similarly, the involuntary muscles are first developed and afterwards the voluntary.

† The difference between these nerves is very remarkable on the application of galvanism; for, whilst we found that the voluntary

The points of dissimilarity just now instanced evidently shew that the ganglia and their numerous distributions form an independent system in the animal economy; and that as one thing cannot be said to form a part of another thing from which it is essentially different, so the ganglia and their ramifications cannot be supposed to form a part of the nervous system of animal life, or that which presides over the intellectual and locomotive functions.

The independence of the ganglial system may be farther demonstrated in many of the lower animals, and in the young of the most perfect animals, for in these both the brain and spinal chord may be destroyed gradually; and, provided the function of respiration be not entirely put a stop to, the functions of circulation and secretion will still be continued.

That the independence of this system, and the extent of the peculiar influence which it exerts in the

nerves could be excited with a few plates, two hundred could produce only a slightly perceptible effect upon the parts more immediately supplied with fibrilæ from the semilunar ganglion. When galvanism was applied to this ganglion itself in the recently killed animal, but little appreciable effect was produced either on the vessels with which it is so intimately connected, or upon the stomach and upper portion of the small intestines. In the majority of instances, however, these parts seemed to be in a more contracted state while under the galvanic influence. When the influence of the battery (of two hundred plates) was directed upon the semilunar ganglion of a young cat, it evinced symptoms of pain and distress, and several irregular contractions of the diaphragm supervened. The effects of galvanism were also tried on some of the other ganglia, but they evinced no appearance of being oppressed by it in the dead subject; and in the living the result was equivocal.

animal economy, is farther proven in the most perfect animals, by the effects of disease upon the brain and spinal marrow, either of which may be destroyed to a very great extent, and those organs only which they supply be deprived of their functions, while those viscera which receive the ramifications of the ganglial system will continue to perform their actions without evincing much disorder, unless that part of the nervous mass, which actuates the contraction of the respiratory muscles, becomes involved in the disease.

The ganglia supply with fibrilæ all the organs of digestion, assimilation, circulation and secretion.

The heart is chiefly supplied with nerves coming directly from this class of nerves.

These nerves form a closely reticulated envelope around the arteries of the thorax and abdomen, and around the vena portæ: they may be traced in the larger branches of arteries of the extremities and of the head, until they reach the brain itself.

The arteries throughout the body, and indeed all the other parts of the vascular system, receive nerves directly from no other source than from the ganglia.

The same system supplies, in a demonstrable manner, all the involuntary muscles, and it seems to send fibrilæ to several of the voluntary muscles, especially to those about the centre of the body. It is also liberally distributed to all the secreting glands and surfaces.*

* If, therefore, these nerves are every where demonstrable in the centre of the system, and even throughout its radius, until we arrive

From the manner in which the ganglial nerves invest the arteries proceeding into the brain, and reasoning from analogy, we infer that they accompany the arteries throughout the substance of this viscus; as in other organs of the body, and that they influence its vascular functions in a similar manner.

The chief origin or centre of the ganglial system is generally situated, in all the higher orders of animals especially, about the middle of the body, and, under the name of the semilunar ganglion, it sends off branches which form plexuses; these present modified characters, as respects their external appearance and conformation, in their course to the different organs which they supply.

This central ganglion more immediately supplies

at the superficies or extreme parts of the body, where it may be supposed that they must elude, from the nature of their organisation, the detection of the senses, it cannot be contrary to the uniform operations of nature, and to the many analogies she presents, to infer that they are distributed to the extreme ramifications of the arteries, upon whose trunks and larger branches they are readily demonstrable. And if they are also shewn to exist in some voluntary muscles, may they not be considered to be present in all, bestowing upon these muscles peculiar energies, the nerves of animal life producing the functions which usually result from this class of nerves, in addition to those arising from the involuntary influence or vital energy which these muscles derive from the ganglia and their distributions?

It may be mentioned, that, consistently with the opinions we entertained respecting the independence of, and extent of the functions performed by, the ganglia and their distributions, that we assign the terms—ganglial system, organic system of nerves, vital system of nerves, synonymously; and we use the terms—cerebro-spinal system of nerves, voluntary nerves, and sentient system, also synonymously.

the organs of digestion, chylifaction and circulation, where the expenditure of the vital influence is greatest, and sends communicating branches to the subordinate ganglia and plexuses.

The external characters of the ganglia and of their plexuses and ramifications vary considerably in different situations, both as respects their colour, their external form, and internal structure.

The subordinate ganglia, while they seem to receive a reinforcement of vital influence from the centre ganglion, modify that influence, and generate an accession to it, suitable both in kind and in degree to the functions of the organs which they are destined to actuate.

This class of nerves send off and receive chords of communication between the brain and its subordinate organs, and between the spinal marrow and its distributions: this seems to give rise to a reciprocal communication of influence between the organs of nutrition, &c. and those of relation, and a mutual dependence of function, which is more intimate and apparent as we rise in the scale of creation,—the independence of the former class of functions becoming more evident as we descend, and, the younger the animal is, as we ascend the scale.

The extent and mode of communication between different parts of the voluntary nerves and the ganglia and their distributions vary very considerably.

As this class of nerves are so entirely different in their appearance, structure, properties, and mode of distribution, and as they supply very different organs from those which receive the encephalic class of nerves, so it may be inferred that they perform essentially different functions, although these functions, in the higher animals more particularly, are in close relation with those of the rest of the body.

As it is demonstrated, that the ganglial or vital nerves supply the heart; that they surround and are ramified in the arteries throughout their distribution; that no part of the vascular system receives in a direct manner any voluntary nerves; and as it is reasonable to suppose that this provision does not exist without accomplishing important purposes in the animal economy, and as the fibres of involuntary muscles are evidently supplied from the same source; and, farther, as we cannot suppose, conformably to the laws of nature, that the bare coats of the vessels, and particularly of the arteries, without such a provision, could be possessed of any vital properties,—so we infer that all the vital phenomena which the vascular system exhibits throughout the body are under the direct influence of this class of nerves.

The distribution of these nerves around the arteries, and the manner in which their fibrilæ penetrate the coats of these vessels, seem to evince that they not only impart to them whatever vital properties they may possess, but that they moreover produce those changes on the blood to which it is subject whilst flowing in the vessels, and many of those phenomena which this fluid presents soon after it has been taken from the body.

It is also reasonable to suppose, that the influence exerted by this system on the capillaries, and the additional influence which its ramifications bestow on the substance of the viscera, combine to produce the secretions in secreting organs and surfaces, and nutrition throughout the textures of the body. Hence, that the varied phenomena displayed by the blood itself, by the functions of digestion, secretion,* assimilation, &c. result from the condition of the influence

* No experiment instituted with the intention of shewing the influence of the nerves given off from the brain and spinal chord upon secretion, can prove the reality of such influence; because these orders of nerves are not ramified upon the vascular system, nor do they even supply the capillary vessels. This is a wise provision; for if the heart and blood-vessels were directly under the influence of the voluntary nerves in any of its divisions, this system would be constantly deranged by it, and vascular disease be incomparably more frequent and fatal. Such experiments, were they instituted with the utmost precaution, could prove no more than has been shewn by those of Dr. Phillip and M. Legallois, which, at most, evince that the vital functions resulting from the ganglial or vital class of nerves may be influenced, in the more perfect animals, by the destruction of a part of the nervous system with which they have held, and with which they always hold, a more or less intimate relation; and that the same nerves which, during health, have conveyed a natural stimulus to the vital activity of particular organs, may convey an artificial one; and when the natural stimulus or excitant is removed, or the subordinate function annihilated, the operations to which it is requisite, in the highest animals, must languish and ultimately decay.

Indeed it is only reasonable to suppose, that the involuntary nerves, as they communicate with the organic or vital nerves, convey a natural stimulus or influence to the latter, which, if they were deprived of it, after its continued and uninterrupted influx, which this system, in its centre and distributions, is instrumental in generating in the vessels and fluids which they contain.

The separation from the blood of the materials which supply the waste of the textures, or give rise to their growth, is the office of this system, which imparts its influence to, and operates through the medium of the vascular system.

The vital manifestations of veins and absorbents (with the exception of the vena portæ) arise from the distribution of the system of nerves to the minute arterial capillaries supplying their parietes, and to the adjoining textures; and, probably, from the distribution of minute fibrilæ to their tunics—an organization which, although it cannot be demonstrated, may nevertheless exist, and thus the vital manifestations of the venous system may more readily be explained.

The ganglial nerves sheathe the vena portæ throughout its course in the liver; and from the very abundant manner in which they supply this particular vein, from the conformation of the vein itself both as respects its coats and connexions with the texture of the liver and with the other vessels, and from the character of the blood conveyed to and from it,—we conclude that it is through the vital influence bestowed on the vena portæ by the ganglial nerves, assisted by that belonging to the other

the vital functions of the organs enjoying this additional influence would necessarily languish; or even be overturned if the privation took place suddenly and completely.

vessels and the texture of this viscus, that the changes induced in the blood returned from the digestive canal and its allied viscera, and containing a large proportion of absorbed materials, are produced; and that the secretion of the bile results from the same influence, partly as a consequence of these previous changes, and partly as its independent act, exerted both upon the extreme ramifications of the vena portæ and of the hepatic artery, this secretion consequently proceeding from both the kinds of blood contained by these vessels.

That this system of nerves, by means of the influence derived from its principal and subordinate sources and numerous distributions, and exerted upon the vascular system, generates animal heat throughout the body; and that the production of animal heat takes place in a manner analogous to the processes of nutrition and secretion.*

The state of animal heat, like other secretions, will be greatly modified by the condition, both as respects kind and degree, of the vital influence of the ganglial system, and by the state of the blood on which this influence is exerted, which state will have a double operation in modifying the result.

* The experiments of insulating a limb by dividing all the voluntary nerves and arteries excepting one arterial trunk, performed by Mr. Brodie, in order to ascertain the effects produced from the generation of heat in the limb, prove this proposition, and could not fail of giving rise to what was actually observed. For the ganglial or vital nerves supplying that vessel could not be completely detached as long as any of the coats of the artery remained undivided.

It appears probable, from the effects of several agents upon the voluntary and other muscular parts, when applied immediately to the ganglial or vital system of nerves,—from the general distribution of this system to the capillary arteries,—and from the circumstance of its supplying and actuating the involuntary muscles,—that it also bestows its proper influence upon those which are voluntary, and that thus it gives rise in both to the phenomenon of muscular parts usually called irritability; the different manifestations of this property, as it is displayed in voluntary and involuntary muscles, resulting from the accessory supply of the cerebro-spinal nerves which the former class of muscles receives.

That the ganglial system appears to be productive of certain obscure sensations or instinctive impulses (organic sensibility) which are, by means of the communicating branches of nerves between this system and the cerebro-spinal masses, propagated to the latter; and from the influence they there excite, become the causes of several manifestations, which more immediately proceed from this latter part of the nervous system.

This operation of the ganglial system on the functions of the cerebro-spinal system, is more remarkable when the former is influenced by disease or by a stimulus which is unnatural either in kind or degree; or even when a natural excitant to which this system has been accustomed is withheld, whether such excitant operates either directly or indirectly, or in both ways, as the supply of food, &c.

So little are the ganglia influenced by the operation and excitements of the brain, that organic sensibility is only slightly produced by them. If, therefore, the impulses of passion and volition produce but an obscure effect upon the ganglia and their chief centre, it is not to be wondered that the galvanic influence,—which must be very considerable to equal the impulses of volition,—should act comparatively in a very slight and almost insensible manner upon this system.

Irritations of the ganglial system appear to act in a slight and obscure manner upon the voluntary organs, through the medium of the communicating or conducting branches between this system and the spinal chord.

The influence of the ganglial on the cerebro-spinal system is more marked as the development and functions of the former system predominate, as in the lower animals and in the fœtus of those which belong to the highest orders.

As the ganglia of the great sympathetic form an independent system, presiding over certain functions which are essentially vital, consequently they may be viewed as the system and seat of organic life, and may therefore be denominated the vital system of nerves, whose centre is the semilunar ganglion.*

* Violent blows or contusions on the epigastric region, when they do not immediately destroy the individual subject to them, depress in a very remarkable manner the vital energies of the system. The animal heat is uncommonly diminished, the surface is cold and pale,

It seems probable, from the circumstance of a separate ganglion or plexus, or both, being generally assigned to each important secreting or animalising organ, that the centre or source of vital influence does not supply the whole vitality distributed by the ganglial ramifications to the individual organs and textures; but that the vital influence proceeding from this centre is reinforced by that which is produced by the subordinate ganglia, and is not only reinforced, but modified by them, and by their distributions in the various organs, so as to give rise to the specific difference of function which each performs; and that the vital manifestations of particular ganglia are still farther modified by the communicating branches between them and the cerebro-spinal system, the extent of modification being relative to the extent to which the nerves of this latter system either communicate with, or contribute to supply or to form, the individual subordinate ganglia.

The vital influence being thus produced from the centre of the body, and reinforced and modified by subordinate ganglia, allotted to the individual organs, according to their functions, is propagated along the distributions of the system on which it

the pulse slow and scarcely perceptible, and the breathing feeble and very slow. An analogous effect, in some respects, is produced by concussion of the semilunar ganglion, as that which follows concussion of the brain: in the former, the vital or organic actions are either exhausted or destroyed; in the latter, the animal or voluntary operations only are suspended.

depends and is inherent, throughout the whole body.*

* GENERAL FUNCTION OF THESE ORGANS.

From Notes to Richerand—published in 1824.

[Recognizing irritability as combined organic sensibility (unconscious) and contractility, Dr. Copland proceeds as follows:—]

Organic sensibility refers to those sensations which are produced in different degrees of intensity, owing to the existence of certain conditions of those viscera which are immediately subservient to the preservation of the individual and the species—to nutrition and reproduction, and which are not immediately subjected to the influence of volition. The conditions of the parts exciting sensibility are very various, and are the result of irritations arising from the presence of a stimulus, of unnatural actions supervening in particular systems or textures, and of the deficiency of that stimulus or influence to which particular viscera have become accustomed. Many of the changes preceding this class of sensations seem to interest, in the first instance, the ganglial class of nerves; but, owing to the intimate relation subsisting between this part of the nervous system and the voluntary or sentient part, the impression or change is propagated to the brain. This is the only essential difference which exists between this and the other forms of sensibility. It is the brain which perceives in them all; and although stimuli, or the defect of stimuli, may give rise to certain phenomena possessing the characters of the higher manifestations of this property in the organs appropriated to the preservation of the organic system, independently of the sensorium,—consciousness, or the more perfect form of sensibility, cannot form part of the results.

Organic sensibility may be active or passive—it may or it may not be attended with consciousness; and even the unconscious mode of it may indirectly impel to action, or give rise to many of the manifestations or instincts which characterize the lower animals, owing to the ganglial centres, either from their organization or connexions, or from both, performing a greater extent of function than usually falls to their share. If, therefore, the passive form of organic sensibility may propel to action without consciousness, or the sensorial sensibility being excited, in these animals, we may also account in the same manner for many of the instinctive functions being performed when we cannot trace them to the influence of a cerebral organ. Of all the conditions of sensibility, the active organic form is the least under the control of the mental powers. It also, in all its modes of existence, more intimately interests the existence of the individual than the other forms of sensibility,—organic sensibility involves a feeling in all its active manifestations instinctive of life or death.

From this it will be readily seen how close a connexion exists between organic sensibility and the animal instincts.

Contractility is essentially a vital phenomenon, and is the result of a change in the relative position of the molecules composing the solids of a living body. This property may be divided into the following grades.

1. *Insensible organic contractility,* or that usually denominated *tone* or *tonicity*. This grade of contractility is not confined to the animal kingdom; it is the property of vegetables, and of animals not possessed of a heart. It is diffused throughout the tissues. The vascular system possesses it in the most eminent degree; and it may be viewed as the result of the vital influence with which the structures are endowed; it is more or less perfect as the vital energy is perfect, and it disappears with the extinction of this principle. It is a property of the tissues and of the vessels, which is more or less exerted in all the vital operations—in the circulation, the secretions, nutrition, and absorption. The ganglial or organic class of nerves seems to be instrumental in its production and preservation in the animal kingdom.

2. *Sensible organic contractility* or *irritability* is that inherent property of contraction which exists in all muscular and in some other textures. It is excited by the application of a variety of irritants. It seems to depend upon the ultimate distribution of the nervous substance of these parts, and chiefly upon the nerves proceeding from the ganglia.

Both these species of organic contractility seem to result from one species of influence, with which animal bodies are endowed—they are the proximate result of vitality, and merely differ from each other owing to the intimate structure of the parts in which they are seated, and to the extent to which each of the parts evincing their presence is supplied with ganglial ramifications.

3. *Cerebral contractility* is the contraction occasioned by the will in voluntary muscles. [But this is not necessary to our view of ganglionic function.]

The first and second species of contractility result from the ganglial distribution and influence.

Were the Editor to add here still more recent doctrines on this portion of the nervous system, it would be by quoting those of Müller. But, as already said, his invaluable Manual is, or ought to be, in the hands of every student.

DOCUMENTS RELATIVE TO THE NERVES.

THE Editor at first thought of devoting a part of this work to some notice of Papers on the Nerves, and especially on the Trifacial Nerves, in consequence of its having been pretended that the Ganglionic Portion of these Nerves bears some analogy to the Posterior Spinal Roots. But as this pretence arises out of a mere hypothesis, he gladly eschews a subject which has given occasion only to such conduct and such crimination as are very discreditable to British physiology.—He will only add a few words on the absence of all analogy between the nerves alluded to.

The posterior roots of any one spinal nerve arise from one and the same part of the spinal cord; the ganglionic portion of the trifacial is connected with several distinct parts of the brain:—the posterior roots of a spinal nerve are supposed to exercise A SINGLE FUNCTION—*either the sensory or the motory;* the ganglionic portion of the trifacial exercises at least TWO FUNCTIONS—*the sensory and the involuntarily-motory.*

The existence of a ganglion on a nerve is no test of its being a nerve either of sensation or of motion. *There are nerves of sensation without ganglia,* as the olfactory and optic (for the bulbs of the olfactory and the tubercles of the optic, both of which are of cerebral structure, and become hollow in lower animals, bear no sort of resemblance to the knot on the trifacial, which is of fibrous structure and always retains its character); and *there are ganglia on motory nerves,* the iris and the muscles of the internal ear being supplied from the ophthalmic and optic ganglia.

Such loose analogy and wild hypothesis as those here combatted have no other commendation than their *convenience* to the hypothetist, and they certainly would not be suffered in any other department of exact science.

STEWART AND MURRAY, PRINTERS, OLD BAILEY.